# Healthy Haiku 3:

# How to Fight Childhood Obesity One Poem at a Time

## DR. IMANI MA'AT

Dr. Imani Ma'at

## Disclaimer:

Information contained in this series is for information purposes only and is not intended to substitute for medical advice. Nor is the author attempting to recommend, diagnose or treat any particular illness or disease. It is always well advised to consult with your physician or other medical practitioner before starting any major health regimen.

In association with China Berry Tree Books ®

ISBN: 0-9816305-2-9
ISBN-13: 978-0-9816305-2-6

Dr. Imani Ma'at

# DEDICATION

This book is dedicated to My Sister and
Best Friend Arlene Fabio:
It's your time to soar!

In Loving Memory of my dear friend
Elouise Thomas who always encouraged me
to Do Me and avoid the distractions!

Also, In Loving Memory of
the Great Poet and Author
Dr. Maya Angelou
(April 4, 1928 - May 28 2014)

"My mission in life is not merely to survive,
but to thrive; and to do so with
some passion, some compassion,
some humor, some style!"

Dr. Maya Angelou

Dr. Imani Ma'at

## ACKNOWLEDGMENTS

Thanks to:

My Family

Teresa R. Kemp "Nana Efua Adadzewa,"

Writing Mentor Professor Murhl Teresa
Bussey, Master Editor

Nat White, Jr., Master Editor

W. Calvin Anderson (Educator &
Development Consultant) Editing

Brigitte Keane (Dear Friend) Editing

Dave Ryback (GA NSA) Suggested Brilliant
Subtitle

N. Ann Hall (Own Your Idea LLC)
for Editing and Formatting

Calvin G. Sims, Sr.
for Formatting and Revisions

Dr. Imani Ma'at

# TABLE OF CONTENTS

# FOREWORD

The study of Haiku has long been a part of required English Language Arts learning requirements in the U.S. because this form of poetry has strict structural rules and is a popular art form. This language challenge in a fun supportive group concerned about longevity and a healthy life, allows participants to share ideas and to tell stories. During the Healthy Haiku Workshops, participants learn and have fun with all kinds of health and lifestyle issues.

Dr. Imani Ma'at

Imagine creating your own poetry as a result of healthy discussions and ideas about food and nutrition to transmit something very powerful that you can share -- in the fewest possible words. The Healthy Haiku Workshops can target any population of learners requiring new self- reflective practices and healthy alternatives for diet, nutrition, conflict resolution, wellness and long life.

W. Calvin Anderson, Educator

# Healthy Haiku

Dr. Imani Ma'at

## PREFACE

*"Haiku is a poetic art form that originated in Japan in the seventeenth century. It tells a story concisely and with few words, it uses 17 syllables on three lines usually configured as 5 syllables - 7 syllables - 5 syllables."*

We at Healthy Haiku Productions, are dedicated to fostering healthy choices and improving healthier outcomes for youth, adults and families through poetry, dramatic expression, and other therapeutic and creative techniques!

From the first lollipop that we give a child to the ice-cream cones, candy and sugary breakfast cereal that we offer, we send messages to children that equate sweets with love, feeling good, good behavior and/or rewards for accomplishments.

These simple acts start a trajectory of eating sugary and fatty foods when we feel good or want to feel good. Happiness becomes equated with a sweet taste in the mouth.

I love the Healthy Haiku Poetry Series and I believe that it is my gift to the world. It gives us options and fun ways to counter the barrage of sweets taunting children eye-level in the grocery store checkout lane. I conduct Healthy Haiku workshops and provide books containing inspirational concepts as part of my comprehensive program for holistic health and wellness. My focus is on wellness and primary prevention.

I have dedicated my career to creatively teaching ways to be healthy through nutrition and exercise, in order to prevent the onset of diseases such as diabetes, hypertension and more. In addition to this, I offer lectures and luxury retreats to teach participants about the importance of alkalizing the body, natural pain relief and alternative ways for people to achieve homeostasis or balance in their bodies.

Dr. Imani Ma'at

In my training as a health educator and through my twenty plus years working in public health, I learned that the definition of prevention includes: primary prevention (preventing illness and disease); secondary prevention (screening for and early detection of disease and illness); and tertiary prevention (reducing the discomfort and consequences of illness and disease and averting premature mortality).

I noticed that the emphasis was mostly on secondary prevention. This perspective seemed unbalanced – without enough focus on true primary prevention. I also concluded that health care spending is lopsided in favor of secondary and tertiary prevention. My focus here is all about primary prevention.

Through my workshops and lectures, I also encourage youth and adults to find that one particular thing that for this lifetime is unique to them and only them. I support their development by telling them that their journey is one that is specific to them and they must discover that one thing (or gift) that they could share with the world.

I was recently watching some clips of the beloved late comedian Robin Williams – whose gift was to make people laugh and to entertain in a way that no one else in the world could do. He did so in spite of his deep-seated pain, which ultimately led to him terminating his own life.

I offer this series with love and in the hopes that it will have a positive impact on someone's life (many someone's!).

My goal is to inspire individuals to make different health choices that may enable them to develop their gifts for the world. In this particular series are gems — both in the narrative and in the Haiku poetry that are there to help guide nutritional and other health decisions.

Another goal of this series is to educate individuals regarding the importance of eating natural, live and raw foods. The reason for this is because natural, live and raw foods contain the enzymes needed to digest and utilize the foods that we eat. As a result of eating the Standard American Diet (S.A.D.) so many families battle with generational obesity and complications thereof because of the over consumption of dead — de- nurtured foods that are not digested properly.

As a result, dead, de- nurtured foods cannot be assimilated in a form that the body can readily use to create the healthy cells it needs on a daily basis.

In a healthy adult, it is estimated that 1 million to 3 million cells die and need to be replaced every second.

Do not take my word for it. Research it and you will see a broad range of estimates.

In fact, for millions of Americans it is essential to eat mostly fresh fruits, vegetables, seeds, nuts (living foods) daily in order to change their health trajectory. Equally important is alkalizing because many of the foods that we eat and beverages that we drink are very acidic. Simply alkalizing may change the health outcomes of so many people. That is my greatest hope!

Dr. Imani Ma'at

## HOW TO USE THIS BOOK

This book is the third in the Healthy Haiku Productions (HHP) Series of books (http://www.healthyhaikuproductions.com) and the first to be introduced as an Ebook for easy downloading and access. It is designed to do several things. First, it serves as an aid for teachers and mentors. The term "mentor" will be used to encompass all adults who work with youth and are responsible for youth development including all educators and parents who work with youth. It may be particularly helpful to those needing alternative strategies to educate and motivate the underserved and at-risk youth.

Second, this book serves as a guide for: 1) helping children, teens and their mentors explore important nutritional health issues; 2) introducing children and teens to the world of poetry - Haiku in particular, 3) assisting teens in using their creative talents to describe feelings and experiences related to diet and nutritional health issues using a self-reflective process; and 4) creating a Power Source Prompt (PSP) for youth to draw upon when faced with real life challenges regarding their diets and nutritional health.

A PSP, a term that I introduced through this series, is similar to a cue for action from the Health Belief Model of behavioral change.[1]

Many youth in communities across the country encounter challenging situations that test them and force them to make decisions. When a stimulus is introduced, for example a potentially violent situation, the Healthy Haiku discussion and perhaps particular poems and stories may come to mind and serve as a PSP. A PSP is a trigger that takes one back to their power source or inner strength to effectively deal with the potential risk.

A PSP may become a way out of a tough situation regarding peer pressure to smoke, engage in risky sexual activity or consume excessive quantities of de-nurtured - acidic foods and beverages.

The idea is that as a result of participating in a Healthy Haiku Workshop, lessons and experiences gleaned from the workshop will serve as PSP. This theory has been validated via an evaluation process funded by Morehouse School of Medicine, Tuskegee University and University of Alabama, and will be further assessed through additional evaluations of the workshops over time.

As an example, say 9-year old Janet's parents always pack healthy lunches for her. Other children have often teased her for eating fruits, vegetables, seeds and seaweed for lunch. Janet then attends a Healthy Haiku Workshop that focuses on nutrition. She learns how to value her diet and encourage others to consider eating the same way.

Also, if Janet is subsequently teased by her peers for healthy eating, she may disregard their teasing primarily because she has acquired enhanced skills relating to the importance of eating a healthy diet, maintaining a healthy body and speaking up for herself.

She may have written a particular poem in this workshop or she may have read or heard one that someone shared about the importance of fruits and vegetables that supports her position. For this reason, Healthy Haiku workshops are informative, fun and educational. The workshops can in turn change the mindset of the youth by aiding him or her in making decisions regarding healthy eating as a normative behavior based on their own words and experiences.

Dr. Imani Ma'at

Mentors play an important role in communicating concepts, ideas, and values to youth. Because an effective mentor can have a life-changing impact on a young person, he or she can positively change the course of a young person's life. Overall, this workbook provides handy tools and references to create dialogue with youth about diet and nutritional health issues and about stepping into their power in terms of their health to become all that they can be in this lifetime.

The book begins with information that provides an in-depth look at the consequences of childhood obesity. Included are examples of relevant Haiku and some original poems (non- haiku). Subtext follows most of the Haiku poems in parentheses and italics.

XXX

This is just one of several interpretations provided to stimulate participants mentally and to promote discussion.

There is a "Notes to Myself" section at the end of each page, which provides space for Mentors and students to write their own poetry on the subjects.In addition to healthy haiku, the "To Do Box" contains activities that mentors can facilitate or encourage youth to do in their spare time, as well as in the context of the group.

Haiku is taught and encouraged; however, if the form is too restrictive to them, mentors should be flexible and allow young people to express themselves in the manner that is most comfortable to them. For example, some youth may want to write rhyme, rap or spoken word about their topic.

These activities build self-esteem and reduce the risk of unhealthy behaviors while increasing healthy choices.

At the end of the book are questions for group discussion arranged by chapter, to encourage self-reflection and suggested role-play activities that can be acted out by participants in order to reinforce the lessons learned in the chapter. The role-play activities are highly recommended since participants have an opportunity to demonstrate and further develop skills related to the lessons in the book. Mentors can then ask for comments from the role-playing participants about their roles and how effective they thought they were, followed by comments and feedback from the on-lookers.

The recommended way for mentors to use this book is to be aware of the entire series of Healthy Haiku books and to learn what each book has to offer and then select one book at a time to explore.

I highly suggest you review and utilize the Creativity chapter in the Healthy Haiku Training Manual 5 as a "warm-up" module, that encourages youth to "amp up" their creative juices through music, movement, singing or writing about anything. It does not have to be about a health issue.

Creativity is the core of this program. This is what sets it apart from other approaches of teaching health issues to youth.

Just as I have taken creative license with the use of Haiku, mentors should also play with and recreate the Creativity lesson in a way that suits their teaching style as well as the learning styles and interests of the students.

For example, what may be most appropriate for a group of high school students may be free style rapping about any issue that the students select. For a middle school class it may be gathering around the piano and letting a student play (if any can) and singing songs as a group. Lastly, elementary students might prefer drumming and shakeres (African instruments made from gourds with beads draped on them - used for rhythm).

Read the introduction to a large or small group of students. You may also choose to have the students break up into several groups and read selections of poetry in the book. The groups may decide to explore different aspects of nutrition and wellness. For example one group may focus on the nutritional benefits of fruits; another may focus on the nutritional value of vegetables; and another might focus on the negative consequences of eating foods that are not good for you. Each group can decide their focus.

Each group must select: 1) a facilitator to solicit input from all participants and to keep the discussion moving; 2) a note taker or recorder to document the discussions and poems written by the group members; and 3) a speaker (or speakers) who will share the highlights from the discussion and poems with the larger group.

In the small groups, ask the students to: 1) discuss the diet and nutritional health concerns; 2) individually write 2-3 haiku poems in their own words; and 3) contribute to the writing of 2-3 haiku or other poems with their group members. This activity facilitates teamwork.

Engage students and create peer interaction by having them share highlights from their discussion and to orally present the poems in the large group setting.

Mentors might consider having the students videotape the presentations and watch them to observe themselves and self-reflect. This will reinforce lessons learned and support their ability to speak in public by raising their levels of confidence as they become aware of how they present themselves.

Depending on the amount of time available, mentors can choose from several formats: 1) small groups in which the students explore diet and nutrition in detail and create original poems as described above, or 2) each session or month, the entire group/class can focus on one aspect of diet, nutrition and obesity at a time and explore many aspects of that subject.

At the end of each segment, mentors should review the contents of the "To Do Boxes" with the youth and ask them for other suggestions.

At the conclusion of the book, pose relevant questions to the youth. To supplement the lessons, field trips to various educational sites can be planned. For example vegan restaurants, health and wellness centers, relevant performances/plays, etc., can be visited. Mentors should also explore the web sites, organizational contacts and suggested readings at the end of each book in order to add to the lessons offered in each book.

In Atlanta, Georgia, through my work with the teen theater group, Y.E.S. 4 Health, Inc., I have learned that many youth are not sure how to initiate discussion on sensitive subjects - including those related to many aspects of healthy lifestyles.

Dr. Imani Ma'at

The Youth Educational Services (Y.E.S.) 4 Health, Inc. teen theater program, a 501(c)(3) tax exempt not-for-profit organization, was launched in 2002. Y.E.S. is a peer health education program designed to educate young people about diseases and health issues largely preventable through diet, physical fitness, healthy choices, and high self-esteem. The two health issues presented dramatically to date have been diabetes and HIV/AIDS.

> This book can be used by family members and groups to discuss important health issues that may go unspoken until a crisis situation occurs. Being proactive in matters of health is always more powerful than being reactive.

Teens and adolescents often rely on misinformation from friends and the Internet and other sources that may not be accurate or reliable. In Y.E.S. 4 Health, we talked about many sensitive health issues and the students appreciated the opportunity to ask their questions and express their concerns. In addition to group discussions, students sometimes privately approached me or other adult mentors to discuss issues relative to their health. This approach instills the importance of being proactive and nurtures self-confidence. These are major ingredients for ensuring healthy choices and outcomes by youth.

**Learning Objectives:** After studying this book, mentors, teens and others will be able to:

- Describe at least 3 reasons for eating nutritious food;
- Describe at least 3 things that are healthy to eat;
- Describe at least 3 consequences of unhealthy foods;
- Describe at least 3 reasons for alkalizing the body;
- Be able to describe Haiku Poetry form and history;
- Write at least one Haiku poem that describes their concerns about or experiences with overweight or obesity; and
- Identify at least 2 resources that provide more information about childhood and teen overweight and obesity issues.

# Healthy Haiku

Dr. Imani Ma'at

## INTRODUCTION

Like most adults, the average teenager in the United States has a nutritionally poor diet, does not engage in regular physical activity, and may be at increased risk for diseases and health challenges - many of which are related to lifestyle choices and behaviors. Accordingly, disadvantaged youth and/or youth of color (i.e., African Americans, Latino Americans, Native Americans and Asian and Pacific Islanders) suffer disproportionately from diseases and conditions such as obesity, diabetes as well as social health indices such as violence.

As a child, the father of one of my best friends nicknamed me "Fatty Patty." I guess he thought it was cute. I was not fat, but because of his words I have had a "fat complex" all of my life; well most of my life. I think I am over it now. Words are powerful, however, and one of my goals in this series is to use the power of words in a positive and fun way to make people aware of what they are eating while encouraging them to do better.

My heart and motivation is with the children because that is where it all begins. If we can instill a health consciousness in children and teens concerning eating and the positive power of food, then it may potentially last them for a lifetime. Mentors, teachers, parents and others that work with or care for children and teens are my primary target audience.

Bullying and teasing about weight is something that some children are faced with daily. It hurts and it can have long-term impacts. I think that I survived okay. Having a sister that was nearly half my weight further reinforced my neighbor's words to me – that I was fat. But I was also cute, popular, and athletic and his words did not impact me to the extent that they could have otherwise.

Largely due to my parents' encouragement, I was an A student, went on to become Captain of the Cheerleaders and Captain of the Track Team, and played first chair clarinet in the band. I was a leader in every sense of the word.

## The Answer Is Haiku

As indicated earlier, Haiku is a poetic art form that originated in Japan in the seventeenth century. It tells a story concisely and with few words. It uses 17 syllables on three lines usually configured as 5 syllables - 7 syllables - 5 syllables. Matsuo Basho (1644-1694) is the poet who is credited with first writing haiku.[2] One of the best descriptions of haiku that I have read is the following from Dunn Mascetti's Little Book of Zen:

Haiku is like a vortex of energy; a haiku moment is a moment of absolute intensity in which the poet's grasp of his intuition is complete and the image he describes lives its own life. The art of haiku is to frame reality in a single instant that will lock the poet and reader into sharing the same experience. [2]

Haiku is brief, simple and easy to write yet complex. Haiku allows you to share your heart without giving up your soul. What does that mean? It is so brief that it allows you to go only so deep – and then it is over – usually leaving you wanting more even though in most cases you have received the essence of the message. Instinctively you know that there is more and that is where the imagination, self-exploration and creativity kick in. Seventeen syllables, if well-constructed, can open the gateway for an anthology in the mind.

I learned Haiku in elementary school. I thought that everyone learned it in elementary school. Boy was I wrong. I have many adults asking me "now what exactly is Haiku?" As a child I read a lot and wrote often – including poetry.

When I discovered Haiku I fell in love with it. As an adult, while taking a Montessori Teacher Training Course, I was reintroduced to Haiku as a learning tool for small children and vowed to use it often and in a fun way.

Traditional haiku contains a "kigo" or a season word, which suggests a season in which the haiku is set. For example, falling leaves may indicate fall, cherry blossoms indicate spring, snow indicates winter, and mosquitoes indicate summer, but the season word isn't always that obvious. I have exercised my creative, literary free will to share this beautiful and crisp style to invoke creative expression among youth concerning nutrition and wellness.

I have chosen to diverge from the traditional haiku form regarding the referencing of seasons; however, students will be informed about the traditional form and through these workshops, provided an opportunity to practice it.

Many historic figures and celebrities including the Dalai Lama[3] have written haiku. I recently discovered that literary giant – Richard Wright the author of Native Son (1940), Black Boy (1945) and many other books and collections, penned over 4,000 Haiku poems.

Here is one that paints a delicious picture of a ripe green, perhaps honeydew melon:

> As the sun goes down
> A green melon splits open
> And juice trickles out.[3a]

I also visited the work of beloved author and first Poet Laureate of Philadelphia, Sonia Sanchez whose primary collection of Haiku poetry is enshrined in Morning Haiku (2010). [4] She so eloquently states:

*I knew when I heard young poets say in verse and conversation: i'm gonna put you on "pause," I heard their haiku nature," their haikuography. They were saying, I gotta make you slow down and check out what's happening in your life. In the world.*

*So this haiku slows us down, makes us stay alive and breathe with that one breath that it takes to recite a haiku.*

*This haiku, this tough form disguised in beauty and insight, is like the blues, for they both offer no solutions, only a pronouncement, a formal declaration – an acceptance of pain, humor, beauty and non-beauty, death and rebirth, surprise and life. Always life. Both always help us to maintain memory and dignity.[4]*

Haikuography! I love it! Okay, admittedly, contrary to the sentiments of Dr. Sanchez, the point of my haiku IS to offer solutions concerning health and wellness – out of a sense of urgency and caring.

When I have an opportunity to discuss this with her, I am sure that she will be okay with my intentions. Here is one of ten haiku that she wrote in tribute to Max Roach (1924-2007) a famous jazz percussionist:

Nothing ends

every blade of grass

remembering your sound.[5]

As in previous volumes in this series, other forms of poetry are dispersed throughout this book in order to give the reader a variety of poetic expression types. I encourage all forms of artistic expression and all types of poetry, including the current hip-hop genre of spoken word.

# Healthy Haiku

Dr. Imani Ma'at

## HAIKU, HIP-HOP AND SPOKEN WORD

For tweens (those double digit years from 10-12 before age 13) and teens connecting haiku, hip-hop and spoken word can serve as an invaluable bridge to communication and literacy related to healthy options. In healthy haiku workshops, participants are engaged in interactive activities that facilitate team-building skills in addition to literacy competence - related to health and wellness topics. Included in the workshops is a creativity component that encourages haiku creation, however tweens and teens are encouraged to also communicate in a manner that is most comfortable and relevant to them. For many, this means Hip-hop and spoken word.

Numerous educators have documented that hip-hop has had an increasingly stronger influence over youth since the 1990's.

Baker, Farley, and George all argue that the creative people who are talking about youth culture in a way that makes sense happen to be rappers, and the youth are responding in many ways. Hip-hop artists sold more than 81 million CDs, tapes, an albums in 1998, more than any other genre of music. Although Hip-hop got its start in black America, more than 70 percent of albums are purchased by whites. [6]

Hip-hop can be used as a bridge linking the seemingly vast span between the urban streets and the world of academics.

Hip-hop texts can be equally valuable spring-boards for critical discussions about contemporary issues facing urban youth.[6] One of my most memorable experiences with healthy haiku workshops where we included hip hop was at a juvenile justice center where teens who had committed petty offenses were required to report daily after school.

The group was assembled in a circle and was talking about all types of things. One young man, named Michael, unapologetically arrived late - after the session had already started. He was moving towards a chair outside of the circle and I motioned for him to join us. He came over reluctantly and sat with his head down with a look on his face as though – I am here – but do not ask me to participate 'cause I am not!

I was sure that he was not going to participate in any way, shape or form. But as Michael heard the discussion, it drew him in and he started speaking about drugs and homicide (two critical health issues) in his community from a personal perspective. His favorite cousin had started using drugs at age 12.

An uncle, popular in the community was in prison for life for killing a neighbor. Michael poured out his heart that day – and in doing so - emerged as a leader in both large group and small groups where he worked with his peers to write haiku poems and hip hop about their experiences and reported out for his group by reciting the poems to the large group. He approached me after the class, told me he liked the class, thanked me for coming and asked me when I would return.

As he turned and walked away to leave, I believe I saw a tear form in the corner of his eye. For me it symbolized a breakthrough the kind that makes it all worthwhile!

Healthy Haiku Productions has collaborated with and promoted the works of talented Spoken word talents such as Life the Griot (Athens, GA) and Tebe Zelango, (Decatur, IL). The former is one of the collaborators with Healthy Haiku Productions and presented at the annual meeting of the LINKS organization in 2011 with Dr. Ma'at and other team members. The latter is a phenomenal spoken word artist and violinist. Many people say that there are no coincidences or accidents.

I accidentally connected with Tebe because I saw a post on Facebook and was greatly impressed.

His location was listed as Decatur (which I mistook for Decatur, Georgia). I quickly realized that he lived in Decatur, Illinois but feel as though we were meant to connect. Like Brother Life the Griot, Tebe Zelango is a young, talented genius who recites spoken word and plays the violin and guitar - that we want to share with as many youth as possible. I was pleased to have him as a featured artist on the Stepping into My Power Blog Talk Radio Show on September 10, 2013 and grateful that he is now a lifetime friend to me and HHP.

# Healthy Haiku

Dr. Imani Ma'at

## HEALTHY EATING TO PREVENT OBESITY

*"To insure good health: Eat lightly, breathe deeply, live moderately, cultivate cheerfulness, and maintain an interest in life."*

William Londen

As stated in the Introduction, just as the obesity and chronic disease rates are rising for adults in the U.S. many children and teens are beginning to manifest the same health challenges related to being overweight. Sedentary lifestyles are encouraged with excessive television watching and computers throughout the home.

Policy changes that once made physical fitness mandatory in schools, now no longer exist.

De-nurtured, processed foods laden with fats, sugars and salts, are wearing heavily on our youth (pun intended!). Large portion sizes are also contributing to overweight and obese adolescents.

A physician and close friend, the late Dr. Beverly Coleman-Miller, mentioned that while performing autopsies (from gun shot and other non- sickness related deaths), she had seen the insides of many deceased youth. She was alarmed at the amount of plaque around their hearts - the same type of plaque residue on our teeth if we do not brush frequently.

Many of these youth appeared healthy on the outside and were not overweight; however, the damage to their hearts was already apparent.

Proper diets, which include healthy foods such as fruits, green vegetables, grains, lots of alkaline water intake and good fats such as olive oil and coconut are key. These are some of the primary dietary gems in reducing risks for being overweight, obese and developing preventable chronic diseases.

Invariably, when the HHP team of experts holds workshops for elementary school children – when asked to brainstorm on types of healthy foods, the youngest children appear to instinctively know and mention fruits and vegetables as being good for their bodies.

The older children and teens expressed more confusion about what is "good" for your body – often wanting to add foods such as pizza and fried chicken.

Lots of good came out of those discussions, which gave us an opportunity to speak about healthy alternatives such as pizza with whole wheat crust and veggies.

# Childhood Obesity Facts:[7]

- Childhood obesity has more than doubled in children and tripled in adolescents in the past 30 years.
- The percentage of children aged 6–11 years in the United States who were obese increased from 7% in 1980 to nearly 18% in 2010. Similarly, the percentage of adolescents aged 12–19 years who were obese increased from 5% to 18% over the same period.
- In 2010, more than one third of children and adolescents were overweight or obese.
- *Overweight* is defined as having excess body weight for a particular height from fat, muscle, bone, water, or a combination of these factors. *Obesity* is defined as having excess body fat.
- Overweight and obesity are the result of "caloric imbalance"—too few calories expended for the amount of calories consumed—and are affected by various genetic, behavioral, and environmental factors.

Source: CDC. 2013. National Center for HIV/AIDS, Viral Hepatitis, STD, and TB Prevention, Division of Adolescent and School Health and National Center for Chronic Disease Prevention and Health Promotion, Division of Population Health (See references for additional information on primary sources).

In a National Survey of teens, 79.9% had not eaten greater or equal to 5 daily servings of fruits and vegetables during a 7-day period; 67.0% did not attend physical education classes daily, and 13.1% were overweight. [8]

COMPLICATIONS OF CHILDHOOD OBESITY

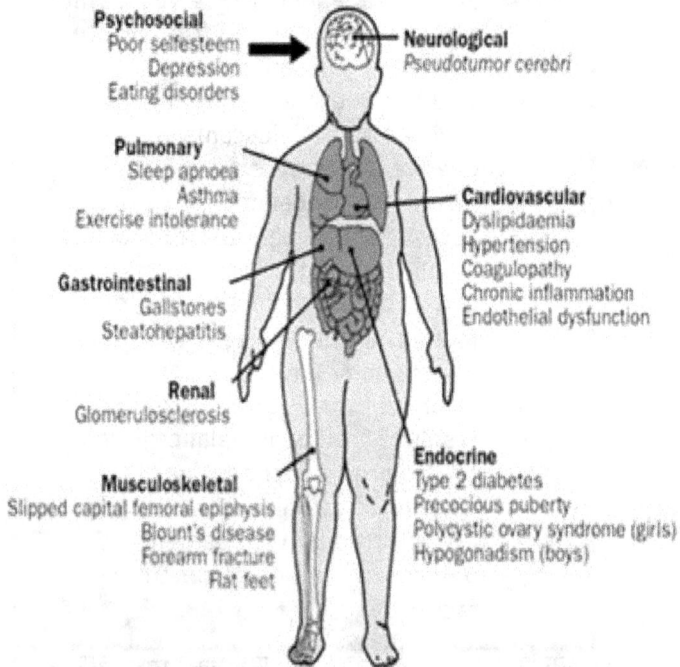

**Psychosocial**
Poor selfesteem
Depression
Eating disorders

**Neurological**
Pseudotumor cerebri

**Pulmonary**
Sleep apnoea
Asthma
Exercise intolerance

**Cardiovascular**
Dyslipidaemia
Hypertension
Coagulopathy
Chronic inflammation
Endothelial dysfunction

**Gastrointestinal**
Gallstones
Steatohepatitis

**Renal**
Glomerulosclerosis

**Musculoskeletal**
Slipped capital femoral epiphysis
Blount's disease
Forearm fracture
Flat feet

**Endocrine**
Type 2 diabetes
Precocious puberty
Polycystic ovary syndrome (girls)
Hypogonadism (boys)

Source: Eaton. et al., 2005.

## THE IMPACT OF OBESITY ON TEENS

The consequences and complication of obesity in teens are enormous as depicted in the above picture. The list includes but is not limited to: diabetes, high blood pressure, heart disease, compromised immune systems, depression and social isolation. According to the China Study (2004), [9] the most comprehensive study of nutrition ever conducted, one of the most important consequences of childhood obesity is that an obese young person is much more likely to become an obese adult, greatly increasing the likelihood of lifelong health problems.

Dr. Robert O. Young and his wife Shelly Redford Young co-authored a book entitled The pH Miracle for Weight Loss in 2005 in which they suggest that we think of our bodies as a Bank Account:

*When you eat electron-rich alkaline foods, you are making a deposit to your account, maintaining an investment in your health, fitness, energy, vitality - and weight. And when you eat proton-saturated acidic food, you are making an energy withdrawal. On the most basic level, if there's not enough in the account to cover withdrawals you're in trouble!...To keep a good balance, so you always have enough energy on hand to draw on as necessary, you need to both limit your withdrawals and make plenty of deposits (in the form of green food, green drinks, and good fats).* [10]

## Diabetes

Type 2 diabetes is a condition in which the body is no longer able to consistently produce the insulin (a hormone) needed to process glucose in the blood. This was once primarily a disease of older adults. It is now swiftly becoming a disease that is impacting many young people due to poor eating habits and lack of exercise. The health risks associated with diabetes are tremendous. Complications associated with diabetes include: high blood pressure, heart disease, blindness, kidney failure, impotence and lower-extremity (primarily leg) amputations.

### What is diabetes?

Diabetes is a disease in which blood glucose levels are above normal. Most of the food we eat is turned into glucose, or sugar, for our bodies to use for energy. The pancreas, an organ that lies near the stomach, makes a hormone called insulin to help glucose get into the cells of our bodies. When you have diabetes, your body either doesn't make enough insulin or can't use its own insulin as well as it should. This causes sugar to build up in your blood.

### What are the types of diabetes?

**Type 1 diabetes**, which was previously called insulin-dependent diabetes mellitus (IDDM) or juvenile-onset diabetes, may account for about 5% of all diagnosed cases of diabetes. **Type 2 diabetes**, which was previously called non-insulin-dependent diabetes mellitus (NIDDM) or adult-onset diabetes, may account for about 90% to 95% of all diagnosed cases of diabetes. **Gestational diabetes** is a type of diabetes that only pregnant women get. If not treated, it can cause problems for mothers and babies. Gestational diabetes develops in 2% to 10% of all pregnancies but usually disappears when a pregnancy is over. **Other specific types of diabetes** resulting from specific genetic syndromes, surgery, drugs, malnutrition, infections, and other illnesses may account for 1% to 5% of all diagnosed cases of diabetes.

Source: CDC. (2012). Basics Facts About Diabetes. [11]

In Y.E.S. 4 Health, Inc, we always try to keep it real.

When teaching the youth in our teen theater program about diabetes, one of the students in our group volunteered to demonstrate the insulin pump that she wore on her waist. She had Type I Diabetes from birth and was eager to demonstrate the insulin pump providing her body what it needed in terms of insulin for handling the processing of glucose (sugar) in her body.

There is a general misconception that diabetes "runs in the family." For some reason this fallacy has made it to the youngest of family members. When speaking to elementary school students, I often ask if they know anyone that has diabetes. Most hands go up in the air.

Many of them think that diabetes "runs in their families" and that they will eventually get it to.

They see grandmothers, aunts, cousins and relatives with diabetes and figure that it is inevitable that they too will eventually become diabetic (or someone told them that). If everyone in the family is eating diets high in processed foods, salts, sugars, fats etc, the same outcome is inevitable. One of the things that we teach in Healthy Haiku Workshops is that we are in charge of our health to the extent that we control what we eat and how much exercise we get.

While it is true that genetics plays a small (very small) role in the development of type II diabetes, most cases are due to eating and lifestyle choices. What appears to run in families is actually shared eating and behavior habits in families that manifest the same results. A good friend, Ivan Juzang, CEO of MEE Productions, told me that "running does not run in many families!"

The doctors are there for guidance and checkups to provide feedback on how we are doing and to recommend medical interventions if necessary. Holistic and Naturopathic doctors and practitioners are also trained to assess ways that the body may be out of balance and need modifications and/or supplementation to get back on track.

**Diagnosed diabetes in people younger than 20 years of age, United States, 2010**

- About 215,000 people younger than 20 years have diabetes (type 1 or type 2). This represents 0.26% of all people in this age group. Estimates of undiagnosed diabetes are unavailable for this age group.

**Racial and ethnic differences in diagnosed diabetes**

- Compared to non-Hispanic white adults, the risk of diagnosed diabetes was 18% higher among Asian Americans, 66% higher among Hispanics, and 77% higher among non-Hispanic blacks. Among Hispanics compared to non-Hispanic white adults, the risk of diagnosed diabetes was about the same for Cubans and for Central and South Americans, 87% higher for Mexican Americans, and 94% higher for Puerto Ricans.

Source: 2011 National Diabetes Fact Sheet. 2013. [12]

The first program launched by Youth Educational Services (Y.E.S.) 4 Health, Inc. was a Theater Program.

The opening season that commenced in October 2003 included an original dramatic play entitled "Drive-Thru Justice," which dramatized the disproportionate impact of diabetes on African American and Latino American communities much of it can be attributed to fast foods and processed food consumption. In the book Fast Food Nation by Eric Scholosser [13] we learn that:

> In 1970, Americans spent about $6 million on fast food; in 2001, they spent more than $110 billion. Americans now spend more money on fast food than on higher education, personal computers, computer software or new cars.

*They spend more on fast food than on movies, books, newspapers, videos, and recorded music – combined.*[13]

The play depicted the brilliantly planned purchase of a fast food restaurant franchise by a small group of African Americans in order to highlight the health hazards of over consumption of fast foods. In the play, a request for French fries, burgers and soda (i.e., typical fast foods) served in "Sweet Burger's" restaurant was denied to an African American woman and her daughter because of the State of Emergency in Black communities regarding their health. Y.E.S. performed for schools and churches in the Atlanta Metropolitan Area and diabetes conferences including one at the Morehouse School of Medicine - all of which were extremely well received.

The play was reintroduced to audiences with a new cast in 2007. Again, it was enthusiastically received.

Drive Thru-Justice © is being reproduced once again by collaboration between Y.E.S. 4 Health and Sons of a Phoenix in 2015. For more information concerning the hazards of fast food consumption including obesity, read Fast Food Nation by Eric Schlosser. [13]

## High Blood Pressure

Teens who are overweight are more likely to have high blood pressure than those with healthy body weights. Lack of exercise and overeating put additional stress on the heart, which must work harder to pump the blood through the system.

Over time, the heart and arteries can become damaged, leading to hypertension and the other serious complications.[14]

## Causes of Teenage High Blood Pressure

It was formerly believed that underlying problems with the heart or kidneys caused high blood pressure in teens. Further research has shown that teenagers develop high blood pressure in approximately the same proportions and manner as adults. Primary hypertension is the term used therefore for most cases of high blood pressure in teenagers.

The causes of primary hypertension are not clearly understood. Some teenagers appear to inherit the tendency to develop high blood pressure from their parents, while others make poor lifestyle choices, including decreased cardiovascular fitness. This is partly the result of the removal of physical education as part of the regular curriculum from many school systems.[15]

*Obesity produces chronic inflammation and compromised immunity that may increase the susceptibility to inflections. Moderate, regular exercise may enhance immunity, but prolonged high-intensity exercise may impair it.* [16]

The hormonal changes of adolescence can also affect risks for high blood pressure.

For example, the combination of poor diets and not getting enough exercise can affect blood pressure in teenagers. Surges in the sex hormones testosterone and estrogen also play a role in the development of high blood pressure among teenagers.

While the precise roles these hormones play are complex and not fully understood, it has been shown that teenagers who begin puberty at a younger age tend to have an increased risk of developing high blood pressure.[15]

## Compromised Immune System

Obesity alters the immune system. Our immune systems protect us from disease, infection, bacteria, etc.

In cases of obesity, immune cells enter fat tissue and accumulate in numbers proportional to the degree of obesity. The fat cells actually protect the body from acidic cells that if left unchecked can burn a hole through the tissues.

These immune cells play important roles in the development of inflammation. A chronic state of low-grade inflammation exists in obese individuals.

Obesity can also increase the susceptibility to infections. Some studies have shown that obese patients have a higher incidence of postoperative and other hospital-related infections compared with patients of normal weight. Obese individuals have also been shown to exhibit poor wound healing and increased occurrence of skin infections.[16]

In general, this means that obese teens are more likely to become sick and miss more days of school and other routine activities.

## Obesity and Depression

The combination of obesity and depression, in a similar fashion to diabetes, have until recently been considered "adult" health problems. This morbid combination is now recognized as common among youths. Recent data from the National Health and Nutrition Examination Survey estimates that 17% of youth ages 2-19 years old, to be overweight compared to just 5% a few decades ago. Also impacting a large population of youth, depressive disorder has been estimated in 2% of children and 4-8% of adolescents. [17]

In Y.E.S. 4 Health, Inc. we were exploring potential health topics with the youth for study and presentation. Several students brought up the issue of mental health - which was surprising to the adult mentors.

They talked about loneliness, isolation and misunderstandings with parents. One student spoke quite candidly of the physical abuse imposed upon her by a parent and the mental scars that had lingered many years after the abuse.

The documented high prevalence of the combination of obesity and mental health problems is alarming given the health and socioeconomic burdens associated with these problems, and the limited effectiveness of current treatment interventions.

The former Surgeon General Richard H. Carmona, M.D., M.P.H., F.A.C.S, highlighted both pediatric obesity and depression as major public health issues.

Also, in the 2000 report on children and mental health, the then Surgeon General, Dr. David Satcher, emphasized that the recurrence of childhood depression episodes is common and depression "may leave behind psychological scars that increase vulnerability throughout early life." [18]

In 2003, the Surgeon General Carmona testified on "The Obesity Crises in America"[19] that the annual cost of obesity in the US in 2000 was $117 billion dollars, and that obesity epidemics have been followed by pediatric epidemics of type 2 diabetes and hypertension.

Interesting observation that in 2001 the public spent $110 billion on fast foods and the cost of obesity in 2000 was $117 billion dollars. Clearly fast food consumption is heavily correlated with obesity.

## Social Isolation

Youth need to learn as children that they are what they eat and that many illnesses are directly related to what is consumed. Many health conditions and diseases can be avoided with healthy diets and regular exercise throughout life.

When addressed early (in children and teens), it is more likely that health challenges later in life are reduced. I remember as a child that the overweight children were last to be picked for softball teams and other sports games that required picking teams.

The countdown was excruciatingly painful and always had the same outcome. Two team captains picked all of their favorite teammates leaving the same last two or three children till the end. Who wants to be consistently everyone's last choice?

They were also shunned in circles of popular children who had higher self-esteems. The building of healthy self-esteem is one of the objectives of all of the Healthy Haiku workshops and training. Young people can and will accomplish so much more if they feel good about themselves. Conversely, feeling good about ourselves can also help us to make healthier food choices and the amount of exercise in which we engage.

Let us reduce the risks of children and teens (the next generation of adults) from developing diabetes, obesity, heart disease and other preventable diseases/conditions by reinforcing these messages every chance we can.

> *The solution ... is a whole foods, plant-based diet, coupled with a reasonable amount of exercise. It is a long-term lifestyle change, rather than a quick-fix fad, and it can provide sustained weight loss while minimizing risk of chronic diseases.* [9]

While this quote is specific to weight loss, it is also applicable to prevention and maintenance of a healthy lifestyle.

Foods and beverages to avoid or eat only in moderation: sugar, pastries, wheat, ice cream, dairy, meats (including fish and fowl), tap water, sodas, and processed foods.

# Healthy Haiku

Dr. Imani Ma'at

## IMPORTANCE OF ALKALIZING THROUGH DIET AND WATER

Seven days a week, 365 days per year, our body fluids need to be at a pH (which stands for potential of hydrogen or power of the hydrogen) of 7.365 on a pH scale of 1-14. Any higher or lower our bodies fall out of a state of homeostasis (pH balance). Homeostasis is the state of being in balance so that the body can function consistently at an optimal level. (Lower numbers – slightly below 7 means that the body is becoming too acidic.)

Acidity is the root of most prevalent chronic unhealthy conditions, i.e., diabetes, high blood pressure, cancers and so much more. Alkaline foods and beverages are required by the body to stay healthy.

An acidic pH can occur in the body from an acid forming diet, emotional stress, toxic overload, and/or immune reactions or any process that deprives the cells of oxygen and other nutrients. The body will try to compensate for an acidic pH by using alkaline minerals. If the diet does not contain enough minerals to compensate, a buildup of acids in the cells will occur.

The body will also protect itself from toxic acids by bonding to fat cells. The body uses fat to buffer or neutralize acids. The fat cells surround the acids to protect the body. Robert O Young and Shelly Redford Young shared in their book, The PH Miracle for Weight Loss, 10 that alkalizing is in fact the key to weight loss.

*A healthy body naturally maintains its own ideal weight...Restoring balance to your system will create a new level of energy and mental clarity – and allow your body to seek its own ideal weight naturally.* [10]

An acidic state in the body will decrease the body's ability to absorb minerals and other nutrients, decrease the energy production in the cells, decrease the body's ability to repair damaged cells, decrease its ability to detoxify heavy metals, make tumor cells thrive, and make it more susceptible to fatigue and illness. A blood pH of 6.9, which is only slightly acidic, can induce coma and death. [20]

The reason acidosis is common in our society is mostly due to the Standard American Diet (S.A.D.), which is high in acid producing animal products like meat, eggs and dairy, and far too low in alkaline producing foods like fresh vegetables and fruits.

Additionally, we eat acid producing processed foods like white flour and sugar and drink acid producing beverages like coffee and soft drinks. We use far too many prescription drugs, which are acid forming; and we use artificial chemical sweeteners like NutraSweet, Spoonful, Sweet 'N Low, Equal, or Aspartame, which are toxic and extremely acid forming. One of the best things we can do to correct an overly acid body is to improve the diet and lifestyle. [20]

*To maintain health, the diet should consist of 60% alkaline forming foods and 40% acid forming foods. To restore health, the diet should consist of 80% alkaline forming foods and 20% acid forming foods.* [20]

*\* See lists of Alkaline and Acidic Foods in Appendix I.*

Many people turn over responsibility for their health to the health care system. As indicated earlier, we are in charge of our health – starting first with our diets and lifestyles.

The late Dr. Batmanghelidj, wrongfully jailed for his political beliefs in Iran, spent many years healing thousands of prisoners and studying the importance of water in the body while imprisoned.

He actually extended his prison stay - longer than necessary - to complete his research. The result was volumes of information some of which is contained in his book: You're Not Sick, You're Thirsty: Water for Health, for Healing, for Life. (2003). His work focuses on the fact that dehydration is the root of many sicknesses and diseases. According to him:

> ...chronic unintentional dehydration in the human body can manifest itself in as many ways as we in medicine have invented diseases.

> We have created an opportunity for the drug industry to thrive, and have given birth to the current "sick-care" health system, at the expense of people's precious lives and resources.

*The sick-care system survives and thrives when people are continuously sick. This is exactly what is going on now.* [21]

From his book Your Body's Many Cries for Water: You're Not Sick, You're Thirsty. Don't Treat Thirst with Medication (1992) Dr. Batmanghelidj provided a long list of the many uses of water in our bodies.

Here is a partial list:

Water:

1. transports all substances inside the body;

2. enhances the collection of oxygen by red blood cells;

3. accelerates the expelling of toxic waste from different parts of the body that is delivered to the liver and kidneys for disposal;

4. it is the main lubricant in the joint spaces and helps prevent arthritis and back pain; and

5. it is used in the spinal disks to make them more efficient shock absorbing cushions.

(See Appendix F for a longer List.)

For those who are not aware of her, I am delighted to share the work of the late African American physician, Dr. Mona Harrison, - preeminent physician, scientist and scholar who shared her life's research work including the importance of alkaline, bio-available water with the world. Some of her of her key points are provided here.

*(Also see Appendix H.)*

1.  Cancer tumors cannot live in alkaline water. All cancer patients should be on alkaline water, and you and I should be drinking alkalized water so our bodies won't provide an environment for cancer tumors to live.

2. Alkaline water is fantastic for insomnia and colic.

3. The brain is 90% water and when it cannot maintain that percentage it will pull water from all other parts of the body.

4. Salt, caffeine, nicotine, Valium, alcohol and sugar put your body out of balance. If we don't keep our blood pH at 7.3 or above, death will occur. In fact, death will occur if the blood pH goes below 7. [23]

Perhaps the best way to explain the power of alkalized bio-available water, is not to tell of the vast number of persons that had been helped with cancer, diabetes, high blood pressure and other health challenges in general but to share a specific story of one person.

In Atlanta, and I imagine in many cities and towns across the country, one of the biggest booming businesses is that of dialysis clinics. Kidney or renal failure is on the rise in communities of color as well as the general population primarily because of our diets and lifestyles. The main purpose of the kidneys is to filter and reprocess the blood.

Specifically,

*Wastes and extra water are removed to become urine, which flows from the kidneys to the bladder to be excreted whenever we feel the need to urinate. But the normal proteins and cells of the bloodstream that we need are returned back to the blood. In this way, the kidneys regulate the body's levels of many substances, sometimes keeping them to a very narrow, normal range....The kidneys release three hormones: one that stimulates the bone marrow to produce red blood cells, another that helps regulate blood pressure, and the third is actually the active form of vitamin D, which helps maintain calcium levels.* [24]

The story is of a relative of mine who is a surviving former dialysis patient of 23 years. That in and of itself (23 years on dialysis) is something of a miracle as he indicated that the average dialysis patient experiences higher morbidity and mortality rates than persons not on dialysis. In any case, he started drinking small amounts of alkalized water in year 21 of dialysis.

People on dialysis are also on liquid restriction so he was limited in the amount of water he could drink on a daily basis. With just small amounts daily, his acne cleared up. He had been suffering from excessive acne from his teen years. In fact, he believes that the medicine that he took for acne as a teen eventually lead to the malfunctioning of his kidneys.

After about 2 months of drinking the alkalized water, changing nothing else in his daily regiment, he noticed a small trickle of urine – he had not urinated on his own in ten years. Hope was restored as he started to urinate on a regular basis – not a full stream, but it was occurring with regularity.

His dialysis routine up to that point consisted of 4 hours a day 3 times a week or 12 hours weekly. Because of his progress, once adding the alkaline water to his daily regiment, while not specifically crediting the water for his improvement, the doctors at his dialysis clinic determined that his kidneys were functioning at a higher level than before the introduction of the alkaline water.

They therefore reduced his dialysis time requirement by 25%. He eventually elected to have a kidney transplant and is doing quite well now at the age of 57. He is writing his own story so I intentionally left out many details of his ordeal. The point is, that for him, alkalized water seems to have played a significant role in his road to recovery and his very existence today.

## What You Need to Know About Enzymes

*Everything that happens in the body - from taking a breath in order to supply oxygen to the blood, to digesting food and then combining digested foods with oxygen in order to produce energy – hundreds of processes require enzyme activity.*

What you should know about enzymes is so important that I have added this brief section to introduce it to many and to serve as a reminder for those that know. Dr. Hiromi Shinya is the esteemed gastroenterologist and inventor of the colonoscopy procedure, which allowed him to remove polyps without potentially damaging surgery through the walls of the colon.

He describes enzymes as being "a generic" term for a protein catalyst that is made within the cells of living things. Wherever there is life, whether in plants or animals, enzymes always exist." He further explains *"enzymes take part in all actions necessary to maintain life, such as synthesis and decomposition, transportation, excretion, detoxification and supply of energy."* He states therefore *"Living things would not be able to sustain life without enzymes."* [26]

There are three types of enzymes: metabolic, digestive and food. Metabolic enzymes operate in all of the cells, tissues and organs of the body; digestive enzymes (three types) – Amylases are enzymes that digest carbohydrates, lipases that digest fats, and proteases that digest protein (Wolfe, 2000). Food enzymes are contained in live and raw foods and are destroyed at temperatures above 118 degrees Fahrenheit.

David Wolfe (2000) a prominent live and raw food expert and advocate indicated that food enzyme shortages sooner or later, result in physical degeneration and disease. When the digestive enzymes present in the body are insufficient, the body draws upon its reserves of metabolic enzymes from the major and minor organs and glands, weakening one's overall vitality.

It takes 10 metabolic enzymes to form one digestive enzyme. Wolfe further states that: "Just because the dangerous effects of cooked and processed foods are not felt immediately does not mean they are not damaging." [27]

The "unfinished bridge" metaphor by Queen Afua, author, health and wellness expert and healer clearly depicts the cycle of poor health and poor health choices by the masses in this country. Read it and weep – or let it be a catalyst for change!

*From cradle to grave, our vital signs tell us something is wrong. Obesity, kidney disease, fibroids, depression, migraines – all clear signals warning us that our lives are out of balance. We have veered off course. We are heading the wrong way.*

*Our path is like an unfinished bridge that sends a steady flow of cars plunging straight into the water. But the cars just keep coming. Each morning, we wake up, start the ignition and drive toward the bridge without pausing to think about the possibilities of a new direction.* [28]

Young people must be confident in knowing that there are indeed options for living a healthy life and for new possibilities to be discovered and explored! It is my hope that through this information, poetry and exercises that they can step into their power and realize their ability to enhance their health and their health outcomes.

# Healthy Haiku

Dr. Imani Ma'at

## HAIKU POETRY RELATED TO OBESITY

Let the poetry inform and set you free! Encourage the young people to write their own poetry in the blank lines entitled Notes to Myself!

**Eat right, get it straight**
**Or it just might be too late**
**Our time will not wait.**

Notes to myself:
_____
_____
_____
_____
_____
_____
_____
_____
_____

Dr. Imani Ma'at

*(Start a plan for eating right to avoid future problems.)*

**Apples and berries**
**Grapefruits, pears, and blueberries**
**Don't forget the cherries.**

*(These are some recommended fruits for your diet.)*

**Live and raw foods help**
**Stimulate our consciousness**
**To see and be well.**

Notes to myself:
_____
_____
_____
_____
_____
_____
_____
_____
_____

*(There are health benefits of eating live and raw natural foods often.)*

**Diabetes is**
**Striking teens when they are young**
**Let's change this around.**

*(Increased rates of diabetes among teens are alarming and preventable.)*

**Let's not be the next**
**Generation of obese,**
**Sick and tired adults.**

*(Take steps to prevent obesity now among yourself and other youth.)*

Notes to myself:
_____
_____
_____
_____
_____
_____
_____
_____
_____
_____

**Polluting our minds**
**Short-circuiting our lives with**
**Fast food disasters.**

*(There are negative consequences of*
*excessive fast food consumption.)*

**Age 4 discovered**
**Mango's sweet succulent taste**
**While in Jamaica**

*(My introduction to mangoes serves as a*
*life-long memory!)*

Notes to myself:
_____
_____
_____
_____
_____
_____
_____
_____
_____
_____

**Don't be blinded by**
**The fancy packaging that**
**Has no nutrition.**

*(Look for nutrition in the foods you*
*consume.)*

**The U.S. is on**
**A crash course of failing health**
**Due to our big mouths.**

*(Do not eat so much & reduce your portion*
*size.)*

Notes to myself:
_____
_____
_____
_____
_____
_____
_____
_____
_____
_____

Dr. Imani Ma'at

**Hiking the mountain**
**Clears my mind and helps me breathe**
**Come hike with me friend.**

*(Go mountain climbing for good health.)*

**Turn off those TVs**
**Go out and play, run, jump, dance**
**Give real life a chance.**

*(Get out and have fun while moving your body.)*

Notes to myself:

_____
_____
_____
_____
_____
_____
_____
_____
_____
_____

**Running low? Running
Slow? Pick up your pace with foods
That ignite your brain.**

*(Eat healthy foods to increase energy and
support the brain.)*

**Trampoline of mine
Exercise body and mind
Fresh air and sunshine.**

*(Personal trampoline (rebounder) is great
exercise and helps to clean lymph nodes.)*

Notes to myself:
_____
_____
_____
_____
_____
_____
_____
_____
_____
_____

Dr. Imani Ma'at

**Burgers and fries just**
**Reinforce the lies they would**
**Like me to believe.**

*(Look for healthier food options.)*

**Chlorophyll from plants**
**Deodorizes inside**
**Your body and out.**

*(If your insides are green; your insides are*
*clean.)*

Notes to myself:
_____
_____
_____
_____
_____
_____
_____
_____
_____
_____

**Overweight and sad**
**Bad things make me want to scream**
**I'll stuff my face glad.**

*(Binge eating out of frustration is risky.)*

**What would life be if**
**There were no Apples to eat?**
**My all-time best Treat!**

*(An apple a day – still keeps the doctor*
*away! Ase')*

Notes to myself:
_____
_____
_____
_____
_____
_____
_____
_____
_____
_____

Dr. Imani Ma'at

**Lemon water it**
**Really "oughtta" be the first**
**Thing you drink each day**

*(A gentle alkaline flush with lemon water is*
*a great way to start the day!)*

**Watermelon and**
**Honeydew cantaloupe is**
**Combined best for you.**

*(Food combining rule: Melons- eat them*
*alone or leave them alone!)*

Notes to myself:
_____
_____
_____
_____
_____
_____
_____
_____
_____
_____

**More protein in Greens**
**Than red meats which are quite lean**
**Just what do you mean?**

*(It is true. Don't believe the lie that there is*
*more protein in meats than veggies.)*

**The closer it is**
**to how it grows —the better**
**it is for my heart!**

*(Heart health begins with nature).*

Notes to myself:
_____
_____
_____
_____
_____
_____
_____
_____
_____
_____

Dr. Imani Ma'at

# RHYMING HAIKU FOR YOUNGER CHILDREN

**Fruit**

I love my apples
Red and green and yellow too!
So healthy for you!


Organic orange
Please make my day in a way
That brings a big smile!

Notes to myself:
_____
_____
_____
_____
_____
_____
_____
_____
_____
_____

Dr. Imani Ma'at

**Strawberries bumpy**
**Blue berries are truly smooth**
**Tell all the good news!**


**A burst of flavor**
**In my mouth - must be cherries**
**Or the Blackberries ~**

Notes to myself:
_____
_____
_____
_____
_____
_____
_____
_____
_____
_____

Cantaloupe melon
Just brings such joy to my lips
As a juice we sip!

Bananas are great
Alone and in cereal
I just cannot wait.

Notes to myself:
_____
_____
_____
_____
_____
_____
_____
_____
_____
_____

Dr. Imani Ma'at

**Tangerines easy**
**Just peel them using your spoon**
**Have one more at noon~**


**I like to eat pears**
**With my big brown Teddy bear**
**In my small blue chair.**

Notes to myself:
_____
_____
_____
_____
_____
_____
_____
_____
_____

**Mangoes, mangoes where**
**Have you been all of my life**
**Always sweet and ripe!**

Notes to myself:
_____
_____
_____
_____
_____
_____
_____
_____
_____
_____

Dr. Imani Ma'at

## Vegetables

**She loves broccoli**
**He loves cucumbers better**
**Greens inside are great!**

**Celery is green**
**Cilantro helps makes me grow**
**So do my snap beans!**

Notes to myself:
_____
_____
_____
_____
_____
_____
_____
_____
_____

Beets are such a treat
Red and sweet we love to juice
Happy as a moose!


Carrots, pumpkins
Very good - so orange too
Sweet peppers for you!

Notes to myself:
_____
_____
_____
_____
_____
_____
_____
_____
_____

Dr. Imani Ma'at

**Nuts and Seeds**

> **Peanut butter please**
> **You can be such a big tease**
> **Protein helps my knees!**


> **Healthy milks for you!**
> **Sometimes flax seed milk will do**
> **Drink almond milk too!**

Notes to myself:
_____
_____
_____
_____
_____
_____
_____
_____
_____
_____

Cashews and peanuts
Macadamia galore
Makes me just want more.


Sugar is sweet but
Makes our bodies so weak and
Honey makes us strong!

Notes to myself:
_____
_____
_____
_____
_____
_____
_____
_____
_____
_____

Dr. Imani Ma'at

# Watermelons with
# Seeds are best forget the rest
# Only real ones heal!

Notes to myself:
_____
_____
_____
_____
_____
_____
_____
_____
_____
_____

## Grains

I ate some oatmeal
Cinnamon and agave
I am not sorry!


So sweet is brown rice
It's natural and healthy
With beans it's so nice

Notes to myself:
_____
_____
_____
_____
_____
_____
_____
_____
_____

Dr. Imani Ma'at

## ADDITIONAL HAIKU HEALTH POEMS FOR ALL

**People get sick hearts**
**Because of what they pick to**
**Eat – We must be smart!**

**A dove above me**
**Sings that there is love around me**
**Starting with good food.**

Notes to myself:
_____
_____
_____
_____
_____
_____
_____
_____
_____
_____

Dr. Imani Ma'at

**Jump up high to the
Sky – water helps me to move
And keeps my skin smooth!**

**The sun warms my toes
I have to breathe through my nose
My heart always knows.**

Notes to myself:

_____
_____
_____
_____
_____
_____
_____
_____
_____
_____

**My daily flax seeds**
**In the almond milk smoothie**
**Provides great fiber!**

**Chia seeds in a**
**Green smoothie adds nutrition**
**In a healthy way.**

Notes to myself:
_____
_____
_____
_____
_____
_____
_____
_____
_____
_____

Dr. Imani Ma'at

**Arise with lemon**
**Water to gently cleanse and**
**Prepare for the day.**

**Fruit for breakfast is**
**An amazing powerful**
**Way to start your day.**

Notes to myself:
_____
_____
_____
_____
_____
_____
_____
_____
_____
_____

# Sweet potatoes are
# Amazing for their fiber
# Taste and nutrients.

Notes to myself:

_____
_____
_____
_____
_____
_____
_____
_____
_____

Dr. Imani Ma'at

## CONCLUSION

This book is designed to provide information and strategies for mentors, teachers, parents and others concerned about the health of young people to share with youth; and to serve as the spark to turn on the "health light" or Power Source Prompt (PSP) in youth who are brilliant by design - from birth. The haiku and other poetry are meant to serve as platforms for discussion, dialogue and creativity leading ultimately to informed choices that reduce risks associated with unhealthy and uninformed choices.

The topics in this volume are very serious and educators and mentors often seek tools and guidance to teach and instill healthy behaviors and decision- making in youth.

This workbook and the workshop series are meant to be such tools that teaches in ways that are fun, interactive, and hold promise for providing lessons that aid youth in their health behaviors and decision-making.

As a Behavioral Scientist, I know that changing behaviors is a process and that people go through stages of readiness before truly committing to and making lasting changes.[29] Reading and studying books such as the Enzyme Factor by Dr. Hiromi Shinya (2011), The China Study by Campbell & Campbell (2005), You're Not Sick, You're Thirsty: Water for Health, for Healing and for Life by F. Batmanghelidj (2003) and all of Queen Afua's books- can greatly improve one's understanding of what it takes to truly achieve optimal health and wellness.

As a quick review, mentors are encouraged to use all of the suggestions from the book and 1) provide an overview of this health issue; 2) read through the haiku and other poetry with the youth; 3) break up into small work groups to discuss and explore different aspects of the health issue; 4) encourage the youth to write their own poetry; 5) review the "To do" Box; 6) use the questions at the end of the book to guide further discussion; and 7) have students perform role-play activities.

Mentors can also take relevant trips in the community to reinforce the lessons learned in the book. Experts may be invited to give a presentation about the topics included in this volume (as well as other topics of interest).

Finally mentors should encourage teens and adolescents to keep track of their growth and development regarding healthy choices. Students should also highlight health decisions that make them feel good (i.e., eating a piece of fruit instead of a candy bar). Responses to the questions, challenging situations, and any discussions or poetry that serve as a Power Source Prompt should be noted in journals as well. Please fill out the Mentor Evaluation form and return it to me. All feedback is critical to improving this volume and making future editions as useful as possible to both mentors and students.

I close with one of my favorite poems that I penned many years ago. "When Spirits Touch" (contained in books 1 and 2 of the series) was inspired by the notion that as spiritual beings living a human experience, we come in contact with other "spirits" on a regular basis.

It could be the acknowledgement of your being by a grandmother who smiles and nods at you in the supermarket (actually happened and served as the inspiration for this poem) or the infant in a carriage who acknowledges your presence even if the parents do not. Whether it is a smile from a total stranger or someone close to you, enjoy those precious moments in time!

Dr. Imani Ma'at

# WHEN SPIRITS TOUCH

When spirits touch
There's a spark
That ignites the soul–
Out of control.

When spirits touch
There's a warmth and a glow
And an inside smile.

Cartwheels of the heart
Jump-start of adrenalin.

When spirits touch
No words of validation
Are needed
To speak what the heart has
Long since connected as real.

**Whether for a moment or**
**For a lifetime.**

**It inevitably lasts for a lifetime**
**Because when spirits touch...**
**There's no taking it back!**

**To Do Box:**

Suggestions to share with young people and their families to reduce their risk for being overweight and obese:

- Ride your bike
- Participate in sports programs
- Swim
- Take long walks
- Eat more fruits, vegetables, nuts, seed and grains.
- Eat smaller portions
- Avoid fast foods
- Reduce fat, sweets, and starches intake
- Avoid soft drinks
- Drink plenty of alkaline water
- Take your parents hiking (i.e., in Atlanta you can hike up the Stone Mountain trail)
- Watch fewer hours of television

# Healthy Haiku

Dr. Imani Ma'at

# REFERENCES

1. Rosenstock, I. (1974). Historical origins of the health belief model. Health Education Monographs. Vol. 2 No. 4.

2. Dunn Mascetti, Manuela ed. (2001). The little book of Zen. New York: Barnes and Noble Inc. by arrangement with The Book Laboratory, Inc.

3. historic figures and celebrities: https://www.wattpad.com/1442693-haiku-quotes-~-famous-people-dalai-lama.

   a. (Source: http://www.ahapoetry.com/pp1 200.htm)

4. Sanchez, Sonia (2010). Morning Haiku. Massachusetts: Beacon Press.

5. Ma'at, Imani (2008) Promoting Health Attitudes, Beliefs and Behaviors Using Haiku and Creative Expression: A Training Manual for Mentor, Atlanta: Focused Health, LLC

6. Morrell, Ernest and J. M. R. Duncan-Andrade, Promoting Academic Literacy with Urban Youth through Engaging Hip-hop Culture. National Council of Teacher's of English. July 2002 88:

7. CDC. (2013). Childhood Obesity Facts. Accessed at: http://www.cdc.gov/healthyyouth/obesity/facts.htm

8. Eaton DK, Kann L, Kinchen S, Ross J, Hawkins J, Harris WA, Lowry R, McManus T, Chyen, Shanklin S, Lim C, Grunbaum JA, Wechsler H. (2006). Youth Risk Behavior Surveillance 2005. Journal of School Health. Sep;

9. Campbell, T. Colin and TM Campbell (2005). The China Study. Texas: BenBella Books.2005: 137.

10.   Young, Robert O. and SR Young. (2005) The pH Miracle for Weight Loss. New York: Warner Books.

11. CDC. (2012) Basic Facts about Diabetes. Accessed at: http://www.cdc.gov/diabetes/consumer/learn.htm

12.   CDC. (2013) 2011 National Diabetes Fact Sheet. Accessed at: http://www.cdc.gov/diabetes/pubs/estimates11.htm#3

13.    Eric Scholosser (2002). Fast food Nation. New York: Harper Collins.

14.    Ray, Linda. (2011) Causes of High Blood Pressure in Teenagers. Livestrong.com. Accessed at: http://www.livestrong.com/article/16251 - causes-high-bloodpressure-teenagers/

15.    Weber, Craig. (2013) High Blood Pressure in Teens. About.com High Blood Pressure. Accessed at: http://highbloodpressure.about.com/od/ highbloodpressure101/a/high- bp- teens.htm.

16.   Drake, Victoria J. (2010) Nutrition and Immunity Part 2. Oregon State University. Linus Pauling Institute. Research Newsletter-Fall/Winter 2010. Accessed at: http://lpi.oregonstate.edu/fw10/nutritionpart2.html

17. Reeves, Gloria M., Postolache,T.T., and Snitker, S, (2008). Childhood Obesity and Depression: Connection between these Growing Problems in Growing Children Int J Child Health Hum Dev. August; 1(2): 103–114. Accessed at: http://www.ncbi.nlm.nih.gov/pmc/articles/PMC2568994

18.   U.S. Public Health Service, Report of the Surgeon General's Conference on Children's Mental Health: A National Action Agenda. Washington, D.C.: Department of Health and Human Services. 2000.

19.   U.S. Public Health Service, Carmona, Richard, M.D., M.P.H, F.A.C.S (2003) "The Obesity Crisis in America" on line: http://www.surgeongeneral.gov/testimony/obesity 07162003.html.

20.   Rense, Jeff (nd) A list of Acid /Alkaline Forming Foods. On line: http://www.rense.com/1.mpicons/acidalka.htm

21. Batmanghelidj, F. You're not Sick, You're Thirsty: Water for Health, for Healing, For Life (2003). New York: Wellness Central.

22. Batmanghelidj, F. (1992,1995,1997) Your Body's Many Cries for Water: Your not sick, You're Thirsty. Don't Treat Thirst with Medication" F. (Global Health Solutions Inc.)

23. Harrison, Mona. Lecture: Water, Water Everywhere but not a Drop to Drink. On line: http://waterozworld.net/watch/lectures/mona-harrison- md.html

24.  Oblas, Agnes (2012) The Purpose of the Kidneys is to Filter and Reprocess Blood. Ahwatukee Foothills News. On line: http://www.ahwatukee.com/columns/health_advice/article_0c6b299a-412d-11e1-beb4-0019bb2963f4.html

25.  Gerson, Charlotte and Bishop, B. (2010 new edition) Healing the Gerson Way: Defeating Cancer and Other Chronic Diseases. Carmel, CA: Gerson Health Media.

26.  Shinya, Hiromi (2011). The Enzyme Factor. Tulsa: Millichap Books.

27.  Wolfe, David (2000). The Sunfood Diet Success System. San Diego: Maul Brothers Publishing.

28.  Queen Afua (2008). The City of Wellness: Restoring Your Health through the Seven Kitchens of Consciousness. New York: Heal Thyself Publishing.

29.  Prochaska, J.O and Diclemente, C.C. (1982) "Transtheoretical Therapy: Toward a more integrative model of change." Psychotherapy: Theory Research and Practice. 19, 276-288,

30.  Meyerowitz, Steve (2001). Water the Ultimate Cure. Summertown, TN: Book Publishing Company

31.    Muhammad,Tynnetta (2003) In
       Search of the Messiah. A Master's
       passing, Dr. Mona Harrison, Transition
       into a Vessel of Light. On line:
       http://www.finalcall.com/artman/publis
       h/columns_4/in_search_of_
       the_messiah_br_a_
       master_s_passing_dr_467.shtml

# Dr. Imani Ma'at

# APPENDICES

A.    Sample Reflection Questions by Chapter

B.    Sample Role Play Scenarios

C.    Vegetarianism

D.    Ice Breaker Examples

E.    More Information and Resources

F.    Water Uses in our Bodies by F. Batmangelidj, MD

G.    The Ten Commandments of Good Hydration

H.    Comments & Lecture Notes by Mona Harrison, MD.

I.    Lists of Alkaline/Acid Forming Foods

J.     Important Quotes from Hiromi Shinya, MD.

K.     Mentor's Evaluation

# Appendix A: Sample Reflection Questions by Chapter and Appendices

1. **INTRODUCTION**: How many syllables are in Haiku? In which country did Haiku originate? Name a famous poet that wrote Haiku poems.

2. **HAIKU, HIP-HOP AND SPOKEN WORD**. How can Hip Hop be used in Healthy Haiku Workshops?

3. **HEALTHY EATING TO PREVENT OBESITY**. What are some of the health consequences and diseases that can occur due to obesity?

4. **THE IMPACT OF OBESITY ON TEENS**
Write at least one Haiku poem that describes your concerns about (or experiences with) overweight or obesity.

Appendix C. Name 2 types of Vegetarians

Appendix E. Identify at least 2 resources that provide more information about teen overweight and obesity.

Appendix F. Name 2 reasons why drinking alkaline water is beneficial.

# Appendix B: Sample Role Play Scenarios

- One teen approaches another who is eating fast foods for lunch. The one that is approaching encourages the other to eat more greens, fruits and grains for a healthier body.

- One teen is on the track team at school and encourages a friend to consider joining. The first teen discusses the benefits of physical fitness.

- One teen is sitting at home playing video games when another stops by and encourages the one playing video games to go outside and ride bikes. He or she also discusses the hazards of sitting around too much and provides good reasons for getting active.

- One teen is eating lots of meat with every meal and another who was raised vegetarian talks about the advantages of a meatless or meat- reduced diet.

## Appendix C: Vegetarianism

Some people choose to follow a vegetarian diet, which means they eat mostly plant-based foods (grains, fruits, vegetables, legumes, nuts, and seeds). However, there are several different forms of vegetarian diets:

- Vegans, or total vegetarians, eat only plant foods and do not eat meat, milk, eggs, or animal foods.

- Lacto-vegetarians drink milk and eat milk products, such as cheese and yogurt.

- Lacto-ovo vegetarians include eggs and milk products in their diets.

- Semi-vegetarians may include fish and/or chicken in their diets, but they do

- Not eat red meat.

- Macrobiotic vegetarians emphasize whole grains, especially brown rice, in their diets and include vegetables, soy, legumes, and fruits. White-meat fish may be included. This diet avoids meat, poultry, eggs, and dairy.

If properly planned, vegetarian diets are healthy and can provide all the nutrients a person needs. As a group, vegetarians are less likely to:

- Develop high cholesterol.

- Die because of coronary artery disease (CAD).

- Develop high blood pressure.

- Develop prostate or colorectal cancer.

- Develop type 2 diabetes.

- Be overweight.

**Living and Raw Foods:**

The largest community on the Internet dedicated to educating the world about the power of living and raw foods.

Web site: http://www.living-foods.com

## Appendix D: Ice Breaker Examples

Most of the ice breakers in this section were taken from:
http://www.mwls.co.uk/icebreakers/

## Standard Introductions

The standard course introduction is to go around the room and have the students give a brief autobiography to include:

• Their name

• Hobbies and interests

## Alphabetic Introductions

Each participant is asked to choose a letter of the alphabet. Duplicate letters are permitted. They are given five minutes in which to describe themselves using single words beginning only with that letter. You could award a small prize for the person with the most number of words.

A further optional stage is to ask participants to write down their chosen words on a sheet of paper with their name at the top and display it on the wall for the duration of the event. Others could be asked later on in the event as to whether the words accurately describe the individual.

## Uses for a...

This is the classic brainstorming exercise where the class is presented with an object - such as a brick or a plastic cup - and the group is challenged to write down as many uses as they can think of for the object.

## What if...

This is an exercise for developing creativity.

Ask a question that starts with: What would happen if... and see what responses you get. The first responses will probably be the obvious consequences of the situation, so encourage the participants to come up with more oblique, less obvious, counter-intuitive or seemingly contradictory suggestions.

You could use questions like: "What would happen if the sea level rose by three feet?" or "What would happen if the average world temperature increased by 10 degrees?"

The first answers will be the ones that we have all heard about on television or have read in the newspapers, but it will not be long before you start getting responses like "Some houses would increase in value because they would now be beach-front properties" or "The British Isles would have colder winters."

## Word Hunt

This is another creativity exercise. The group is given a letter such as "e" or "o" and they are asked to write down as many words, which begin with that letter, as they can think of in five minutes. Names and place names are allowed.

## Name Six...

This is a good exercise for building trust and helping team members to get to know each other better. The team members sit in a circle with the facilitator sitting in the middle. The facilitator chooses one of the team members to start and asks the team members to name, in turn, six places that they have visited. The process is repeated with another subject, but starting with the next team member in the circle.

Continue the session with additional subjects. It's best to start with safe subjects like places you have visited and increase the relevance as you progress. Other possible subjects are:

- Things you are good at.

- Things that you find difficult.

- Things that embarrass you.

- Things you like.

- Things you dislike.

## Picture of My Life

Provide colored pens and sheets of drawing paper. Ask the students to draw a picture of who they are and what they do both at work and at home. You will find that people, despite initial reservations, really get into this exercise and disclose more about themselves.

## Mumblers

When it comes to communication it is surprising to learn that as little as 7 per cent of a communication's effectiveness can be attributed to words alone with voice quality contributing 38 per cent and 'non verbals' providing the remaining 55 percent.

Most people will not believe you when you give them these figures which in a way proves the point so rather than trying to argue the point, try this exercise which is also a great deal of fun.

Divide the group into pairs and give one person in each pair a card with a simple task that they should communicate to their partner. Examples of the type of task would be: 'Close the door', 'Open the window', 'Scratch my back' etc.

They can communicate with each other any way they like gestures, sounds, tone of voice with the exception that they can't use recognizable words. The exercise finishes when the task has been completed.

## Counting to 20 game (creator unknown)

Ask the participants if they know how to count to 20. Of course they all raise their hands. Once that is established, you ask them to get in a circle. The object of this game is for the group to count to 20 - one person – one number at a time without giving visual assistance or verbal encouragement. Everyone is asked to shift their eyes to the floor in the circle (not looking at each other). One person starts by saying the number

1. Someone next says the number 2 and then 3 and so on. The goal is to get to 20 as a group. This seldom happens on the first few attempts. You do not go in order of position. This is a game to promote group work – being in tune with each other non-verbally.

If two people say the same number at the same time, the two people have to sit down. The game starts all over with those still standing. The last two people left standing are the "winner" although this simple game is so much fun that the group rarely focuses on the winners. Truly everyone wins by participating. This is a great game for promoting laughter, fun and really warming up! Young children love this exercise (author unknown).

## Ball of String

Everyone sits in a circle. One person holds the end of a ball of string, shares his or her feelings about the event and then tosses the ball to someone else without letting go of the string.

The person who catches the ball repeats the process. Continue until everyone has made a contribution. At the end there is silence and the strings, which are not crisscrossing the circle, are cut to symbolize the end of the group.

# Appendix E: More Information and Resources

Food and Nutrition Information Center
National Agricultural Library

U.S.S. Department of Agriculture
10301 Baltimore Blvd., Room 304
Beltsville, MD 20705
Website: http://www.nal.usda.gov/fnic

American Dietetic Association
National Center for Nutrition and Dietetics
216 W. Jackson Blvd., Suite 800
Chicago, Il 60606-6995
Phone: 800-745-0775 ext. 5000
Website: http://www.eatright.org

American Heart Association

7272 Greenville Ave.

Dallas, TX 75231-4596

Phone: 800-242-8721


"Overweight in Children ARA

Recommendations"

9000 Crow Canyon Road, Suite S220

Danville, CA 94506

Phone: 925-964-1793

Web site:

http://www.americanheart.org/presenter.jh
tml?identifier=4670


http://DrGreene.com


Shape Up America is a high profile national initiative to promote healthy weight and increased physical activity in America.

If you are concerned that you have a child you think may be overweight or obese, or at risk, this Parent's Guide explains how overweight is assessed in adults and children and it describes the essential components of successful approaches to weight.

Web site: http://www.shapeup.org

Teen Obesity Reaching Epidemic Proportions! Web site: http://www.drgreene.com/21_265.html

KidsHealth is the largest and most-visited site on the Web providing doctor- approved health information about children from before birth through adolescence.

Created by The Nemours Foundation's Center for Children's Health Media, the award-winning KidsHealth provides families with accurate, up-to-date, and jargon-free health and wellness information.

Web site:

http://www.kidshealth.org/parent/nutritio n_fit/index.html

The World's Healthiest Foods focuses on the benefits of healthy eating and how foods affect how you feel, how much energy you have and the length and quality of your life. Sponsored by the George Mateljan Foundation for the World's Healthiest Foods, the site includes recipes, menus and articles about the benefits of various foods.

Web site: http://www.whfoods.com

## Appendix F: Water uses in our Bodies by the late F. Batmangelidj, MD [22]

Why Is Water So Important?

1. Transports all substances inside the body;

2. Enhances the collection of oxygen by red blood cells;

3. Accelerates the expelling of toxic wastes from different parts of the body that is delivered to the liver and kidneys for disposal;

4.  It is the main lubricant in the joint spaces and helps prevent arthritis and back pain,

5.  It is used in the spinal disks to make them more efficient shock absorbing cushions;

6.  Generates electro-magnetic energy inside every cell;

7.  It is the bonding adhesive for the structure of all cells;

8.  Prevents DNA damage and makes its repair mechanisms more efficient;

9.  It is the main solvent for all foods, vitamins and minerals and increases the delivery and absorption of the micronutrients;

10. It is essential for the body's cooling (sweat) and heating (electrical) systems;

11. Supplies power and electrical energy for all brain and nerve functions;

12. It is directly needed for the production and delivery of all hormones made by the brain including melatonin

## Appendix G: The Ten Commandments of Good Hydration found in Water the Ultimate Cure by Steve Meyerowitz (2001) [30]

1.      Drink ½ oz daily for every pound you weigh. A 150-pound person should drink 75 ounces, or approximately 2.5 quarts. One glass every half hour is a good rule of thumb.

2.      Avoid Diuretic beverages that flush water out of your body such as caffeinated coffee, soda pop, alcohol or beer.

3.      Drink more water and fresh juices during illness and upon recovery. Illness robs your body of water.

4.     Start your day with ½ of a quart of water to flush your digestive tract and rehydrate your system from the overnight fast.

5.     Drink water at regular intervals throughout the day. Do not wait until you are thirsty. Thirst indicates an already present deficiency.

6.     Get in the habit of keeping a water bottle with you or keep one in the car and one on your desk. Convenience helps.

7.     Make a habit of drinking water. According to a survey, the reason people do not drink as much as they know they ought to is lack of time or being too busy. Decide to drink water before every meal.

8.     Increase your drinking when you increase your mental activity level; your stress level; your exercise.

9.     Drink the purest water available (Author suggests Kangen water).

10.     Perspire. Exercise to the point of perspiration or enjoy a steam bath. Steam cleans the lymphatic system and blood stream. It is one of the best detoxification avenues available to us....Drink more in hot weather.

## Appendix H: Comments & Lecture Notes by the late Mona Harrison, MD, former Director of the International Water Council.

Dr. Mona Harrison received her medical training at the University of Maryland, Harvard University and the Boston University Medical Center. She is the former Assistant Dean of the Boston University School of Medicine and former Chief Medical Officer at the Washington, D.C. General Hospital. She specialized in pediatrics and family medicine. She served as the Director of the International Water Council and was a researcher at Johns Hopkins University. She passed away in 2003.

Through her advanced studies in the field of quantum mechanics and the laws of cellular and biological regeneration of our DNA, she was led to the discovery of the value of water, its physical, psychical and spiritual properties as the key to our rejuvenation and longevity.

Thus she devoted some 25 years traveling the globe and meeting with scientists from Europe, Africa and Asia who were advanced in the discoveries of this new water technology which she made available in her public lectures, which were full of scientific proof and evidence of the effects of this clean, sanitized water source.

Working in concert with special scientists from around the world, she developed a particular kinship with several water experts from Japan who had studied with Russian Scientists in this field. She later became one of the distributors of certain Electrolysis Machines and other special waters with healing properties for humanity. To this end she devoted the latter part of her life's work as a service to humanity. [31]

## Alkalizing Benefits

- Cancer tumors cannot live in alkaline water. All cancer patients should be on alkaline water, and you and I should be drinking alkalized water so our bodies will not provide an environment for cancer tumors to live.

- Alkaline water is fantastic for treating insomnia and colic.

- The brain is 90% water and when it can't maintain that percentage it will pull water from all other parts of the body.

- Salt, caffeine, nicotine, valium, alcohol and sugar put your body out of balance. If we do not keep our blood pH at 7.3 or above, death will occur. In fact, death will occur if the blood pH goes below 7.

- The hydrogen ion is positively charged....[An ionizer]...changes the hydrogen ion into a negative charge. The liver loves negative hydrogen ions. That is why kidney and liver problems can be helped with alkaline ionized water.

- Urine that has a strong odor indicates an unhealthy body. If the body is balanced there is no ammonia and protein in the urine. An over acidic body causes kidney stones and gall stones.

- Cysts are the beginning of tumors, which lead to cancer because minerals are deficient from that part of the body. Cancer is a long period of mineral deficiency caused by an overly acidic condition of the body.

- The kidney, heart, lungs, brain, intestines, mucous and skin are [electrolytic] membranes and need electrolyzed water.

- Ionized water is great for Attention Deficit Disorder as this condition is [caused by] too much rhodium and iridium in the brain. Ionized water calms these types of children.

- Alkaline ionized water allows greater penetration than any other water and thus wrinkles are reduced because the skin is getting the water it needs.

- When alkaline ionized water was used with Alzheimer's patients, just by drinking a gallon a day, their senility problem subsided.

- Alkaline ionized water is the frequency of the pineal gland and thus affects all other glands below the pineal gland. That is why the water can lower blood pressure and blood sugar, shrink an enlarged prostrate, stimulate sex drive, improve vision, improve Multiple Sclerosis and Parkinson's Disease, just to name a few.

- Reverse osmosis water units remove too many minerals from the water that our body needs and is too acidic for the body to help the overly acidic condition.

- Distilled water is neutral, dead water, and has no minerals or charge.

- Alkaline ionized water electrolysis converts the inorganic minerals present in the water to organic minerals, just like plant juice.

- Alkaline ionized water ties up free radicals from attacking healthy cells.

- Also we are aging too fast because we are acidic and dehydrated!

- Alkaline ionized water is the most powerful liquid antioxidant that can rebuild the immune system and is revolutionizing the health industry. Most of our health problems today are caused by an overly acidic condition of the body.

- Read the book, *ALKALIZE OR DIE*, by Dr. Baroody. He endorses ionized water as one of the best and quickest ways to get the body alkaline.

*Source:* [20]

# Appendix I: Lists of Acid / Alkaline Forming Foods

# Healthy Haiku

## Alkaline Forming Foods

| VEGETABLES | FRUITS | OTHER |
|---|---|---|
| Garlic | Apple | Apple Cider Vinegar |
| Asparagus | Apricot | Bee Pollen |
| Fermented | Avocado | Lecithin Granules |
| Veggies | Banana (high | Probiotic Cultures |
| Watercress | glycemic) | Green Juices |
| Beets | Cantaloupe | Veggies Juices |
| Broccoli | Cherries | Fresh Fruit Juice |
| Brussel sprouts | Currants | Organic Milk |
| Cabbage | Dates/Figs | (unpasteurized) |
| Carrot | Grapes | Mineral Water |
| Cauliflower | Grapefruit | Alkaline Antioxidant Water |
| Celery | Lime | Green Tea |
| Chard | Honeydew | Herbal Tea |
| Chlorella | Melon | Dandelion Tea |
| Collard Greens | Nectarine | Ginseng Tea |
| Cucumber | Orange | Banchi Tea |
| Eggplant | Lemon | Kombucha |
| Kale | Peach | |
| Kohlrabi | Pear | SWEETENERS |
| Lettuce | Pineapple | Stevia |
| Mushrooms | All Berries | Ki Sweet |
| Mustard Greens | Tangerine | |
| Dulce | Tomato | |
| Dandelions | Tropical Fruits | SPICES/SEASONINGS |
| Edible Flowers | Watermelon | Cinnamon |
| Onions | | Curry |
| Parsnips (high | PROTEIN | Ginger |
| glycemic) | Eggs (poached) | Mustard |
| Peas | Whey Protein | Chili Pepper |
| Peppers | Powder | Sea Salt |

| | | |
|---|---|---|
| Pumpkin | Cottage Cheese | Miso |
| Rutabaga | Chicken Breast | Tamari |
| Sea Veggies | Yogurt | All Herbs |
| Spirulina | Almonds | |
| Sprouts | Chestnuts | ORIENTAL VEGETABLES |
| Squashes | Tofu | Maitake |
| Alfalfa | (fermented) | Daikon |
| Barley Grass | Flax Seeds | Dandelion Root |
| Wheat Grass | Pumpkin Seeds | Shitake |
| Wild Greens | Tempeh | Kombu |
| Nightshade | (fermented) | Reishi |
| Veggies | Squash Seeds | Nori |
| | Sunflower | Umeboshi |
| | Seeds | Wakame |
| | Millet | Sea Veggies |
| | Sprouted Seeds | |
| | Nuts | |

## Acid Forming Foods

| FATS & OILS | NUTS & BUTTERS | DRUGS & CHEMICALS |
|---|---|---|
| Avocado Oil | Cashews | Aspartame |
| Canola Oil | Brazil Nuts | Chemicals |
| Corn Oil | Peanuts | Drugs, Medicinal |
| Hemp Seed | Peanut Butter | Drugs, Psychedelic |
| Oil | Pecans | Pesticides |
| Flax Oil | Tahini | Herbicides |
| Lard | Walnuts | |
| Olive Oil | | ALCOHOL |
| Safflower Oil | ANIMAL PROTEIN | Beer |
| Sesame Oil | Beef | Spirits |
| Sunflower Oil | Carp | Hard Liquor |
| | Clams | Wine |
| FRUITS | Fish | |
| Cranberries | Lamb | BEANS & LEGUMES |

| | | |
|---|---|---|
| | Lobster | Black Beans |
| GRAINS | Mussels | Chick Peas |
| Rice Cakes | Oyster | Green Peas |
| Wheat Cakes | Pork | Kidney Beans |
| Amaranth | Rabbit | Lentils |
| Barley | Salmon | Lima Beans |
| Buckwheat | Shrimp | Pinto Beans |
| Corn | Scallops | Red Beans |
| Oats (rolled) | Tuna | Soy Beans |
| Quinoa | Turkey | Soy Milk |
| Rice (all) | Venison | White Beans |
| Rye | | Rice Milk |
| Spelt | PASTA (WHITE) | Almond Milk |
| Kamut | Noodles | |
| Wheat | Macaroni | |
| Hemp Seed | Spaghetti | |
| Flour | | |
| | OTHER | |
| DAIRY | Distilled Vinegar | |
| Cheese, Cow | Wheat Germ | |
| Cheese, Goat | Potatoes | |
| Cheese, Processed | | |
| Cheese, Sheep | | |
| Milk | | |
| Butter | | |

# Dr. Imani Ma'at

**Alkaline:** Meditation, Prayer, Peace, Kindness & Love

## Extremely Alkaline Forming Foods - pH 8.5 to 9.0

9.0 Lemons 1, Watermelon 2

8.5 Agar Agar 3, Cantaloupe, Cayenne (Capsicum) 4, Dried dates & figs, Kelp, Karengo, Kudzu root, Limes, Mango, Melons, Papaya, Parsley 5, Seedless grapes (sweet), Watercress, Seaweeds Asparagus 6, Endive, Kiwifruit, Fruit juices 7, Grapes* (sweet), Passion fruit, Pears (sweet), Pineapple, Raisins, Umeboshi plum, Vegetable juices 8

## Moderate Alkaline - pH 7.5 to 8.0

8.0 Apples (sweet), Apricots, Alfalfa sprouts 9, Arrowroot, Flour 10, Avocados, Bananas (ripe), Berries, Carrots, Celery, Currants, Dates & figs (fresh), Garlic 11, Gooseberry, Grapes (less sweet), Grapefruit, Guavas, Herbs (leafy green), Lettuce (leafy green), Nectarine, Peaches (sweet), Pears (less sweet), Peas (fresh sweet), Persimmon, Pumpkin (sweet), Sea salt (vegetable) 12, Spinach

7.5 Apples (sour), Bamboo shoots, Beans (fresh green), Beets, Bell Pepper, Broccoli, Cabbage, Cauli, Carob 13, Daikon, Ginger (fresh), Grapes (sour), Kale, Kohlrabi, Lettuce (pale

170

**8.0** Apples (sweet), Apricots, Alfalfa sprouts 9,
Arrowroot, Flour 10, Avocados, Bananas (ripe),
Berries, Carrots, Celery, Currants, Dates & figs
(fresh), Garlic 11, Gooseberry, Grapes (less      sweet),
Grapefruit, Guavas, Herbs (leafy green), Lettuce (leafy green),
Nectarine,      Peaches (sweet), Pears (less sweet), Peas (fresh
sweet), Persimmon, Pumpkin (sweet), Sea salt (vegetable) 12,
Spinach

**7.5**  Apples (sour), Bamboo shoots, Beans (fresh      green),
Beets, Bell Pepper, Broccoli, Cabbage, Cauli, Carob 13, Daikon,
Ginger    (fresh), Grapes (sour), Kale, Kohlrabi, Lettuce    (pale
green), Oranges, Parsnip, Peaches (less    sweet), Peas (less
sweet), Potatoes & skin,      Pumpkin (less sweet), Raspberry,
Sapote,   Strawberry, Squash 14, Sweet corn (fresh),      Tamari
15, Turnip, Vinegar (apple cider) 16

**Slightly Alkaline to Neutral pH 7.0**

**7.0** Almonds 17, Artichokes (Jerusalem), Barley-      Malt

# Dr. Imani Ma'at

**Extremely Acid Forming Foods - pH 5.0 to 5.5**

5.0 Artificial sweeteners

5.5 Beef, Carbonated soft drinks & fizzy drinks 38,
Cigarettes (tailor made), Drugs, Flour (white,      wheat) 39, Goat,
Lamb, Pastries & cakes from        white flour, Pork, Sugar (white) 40
Beer 34, Brown sugar 35, Chicken, Deer,    Chocolate, Coffee 36,
Custard with white sugar,      Jams, Jellies, Liquor 37, Pasta (white),
Rabbit,    Semolina, Table salt refined and iodized, Tea black, Turkey,
Wheat bread, White rice, White vinegar      (processed).

**Moderate Acid - pH 6.0 to 6.5**

6.0 Cigarette tobacco (roll your own), Cream of Wheat
(unrefined), Fish, Fruit juices with sugar, Maple
syrup (processed), Molasses (sulphured), Pickles
(commercial), Breads (refined) of corn, oats, rice &
rye, Cereals (refined) eg weetbix, corn flakes,
Shellfish, Wheat germ, Whole Wheat foods 32,
Wine 33, Yogurt (sweetened)

6.5 Bananas (green), Buckwheat, Cheeses (sharp),
Corn & rice breads, Egg whole (cooked hard),
Ketchup, Mayonnaise, Oats, Pasta (whole grain),
Pastry (wholegrain & honey), Peanuts, Potatoes
(with no skins), Popcorn (with salt & butter), Rice
(basmati), Rice (brown), Soy sauce (commercial),
Tapioca, Wheat bread (sprouted organic)

**Slightly Acid to Neutral pH 7.0**

**7.0** Barley malt syrup, Barley, Bran, Cashews, Cereals (unrefined with honey-fruit-maple syrup), Cornmeal, Cranberries 30, Fructose, Honey (pasteurized), Lentils, Macadamias, Maple syrup (unprocessed), Milk (homogenized) and most processed dairy products, Molasses (unsulphered organic) 31, Nutmeg, Mustard, Pistachios, Popcorn & butter (plain), Rice or wheat crackers (unrefined), Rye (grain), Rye bread (organic sprouted), Seeds (pumpkin & sunflower), Walnuts
Blueberries, Brazil nuts, Butter (salted), Cheeses (mild & crumbly) 28, Crackers (unrefined rye), Dried beans (mung, adzuki, pinto, kidney, garbanzo) 29, Dry coconut, Egg whites, Goats milk (homogenized), Olives (pickled), Pecans, Plums 30, Prunes 30, Spelt

**Neutral pH 7.0** Healthy Body Saliva pH Range is between 6.4 to 6.8 (on your pH test strips)

Butter (fresh unsalted), Cream (fresh and raw), Margarine 26, Milk (raw cow's) 27, Oils (except olive), Whey (cow's), Yogurt (plain)

**NOTE: Match with the numbers above.**
1. Excellent for *EMERGENCY SUPPORT* for colds, coughs, sore throats, heartburn, and gastro upsets.
2. Good for a yearly fast. For several days eat whole melon, chew pips well and eat also. Super alkalizing food.
3. Substitute for gelatin, more nourishing.

4. Stimulating, non-irritating body healer. Good for endocrine system.

5. Purifies kidneys.

6. Powerful acid reducer detoxing to produce acid urine temporarily, causing alkalinity for the long term.

7. Natural sugars give alkalinity. Added sugar causes juice to become acid forming.

8. Depends on veggie's content and sweetness.

9. Enzyme rich, superior digestibility.

10. High calcium content. Corn flour substitute.

11. Elevates acid food 5.0 in alkaline direction.

12. Vegetable content raises alkalinity.

13. Substitute for coca; mineral rich.

14. Winter squash rates 7.5. Butternut and sweeter squash rates 8.0.

15. Genuine fermented for 11Ú2 years otherwise 6.0.

16. Raw unpasteurized is a digestive aid to increase HCL in the stomach. 1 tablespoon, + honey & water before meals.

17. Soak 12 hours, peel skin to eat.

18. Sundried, tree ripened, otherwise 6.0.

19. Using sea salt and apple cider vinegar.

20. Contains sea minerals. Dried at low temperatures.

21. Range from 7.0 to 8.0.

22. Sprouted grains are more alkaline. Grains chewed well become more alkaline.

23. High sodium to aid digestion.

24. High levels of utilizable calcium. Grind before eating.

25. Alkalinity and digestibility higher.

26. Heating causes fats to harden and become indigestible.

27. High mucus production.

28. Mucus forming and hard to digest.

29. When sprouted dry beans rate 7.0.

30. Contain acid-forming benzoic and quinic acids.

31. Full of iron.

32. Unrefined wheat is more alkaline.

33. High quality red wine, no more than 4 oz. daily to build blood.

34. Good quality, well brewed - up to 5.5. Fast brewed beers drop to 5.0.

35. Most are white sugars with golden syrup added.

36. Organic, fresh ground-up to 5.5.

37. Cheaper brands drop to 5.0, as does over-indulgence.

38. Leaches minerals.

39. Bleached - has no goodness.

40. Poison! Avoid it.

41. Potential cancer agent. Over-indulgence may cause partial

blindness.

20

Source: http://www.rense.com/1.mpicons/acidalka.htm

Note: No claims are made regarding the therapeutic use of this product...Plus, These statements have not been evaluated by the Food & Drug Administration. These products are not intended to diagnose, treat, cure or prevent any disease.

## Appendix J: Important Quotes from Hiromi Shinya, MD. [26]

This is an important book to add to your family collection on nutrition and health.

Your health depends on how well you maintain—rather than exhaust—the source enzymes in your body. I use the term "source" enzymes for these catalysts, because they are, I believe unspecialized enzymes that give rise to the more than 5,000 specialized enzymes that take on various activities within the human body.

Enzymes carry out the function of maintaining the body's homeostasis — the balance necessary for a healthy life.

Once you clearly understand what exhausts source enzymes and how source enzymes can be supplemented, then, with just a little effort on a daily basis, you will be able to live out the rest of your natural life span without getting sick.

None of my patients have had to face cancer again. Why? Because my cancer patients take their health condition seriously, place their full faith in supporting their body's healing, and practice my dietary health lifestyle daily.

Eating meat may accelerate growth, but it will also speed up the aging process.

## 6 Reasons Why High Protein Diets Will Harm Your Health:

1. Toxins from meat breed cancer cells.

2. Proteins Cause Allergic Reactions.

3. Excess Protein Stresses Liver and Kidneys.

4. Excessive Intake of Protein Causes Calcium Deficiency and Osteoporosis.

5. Excess Protein Can Result in a Lack of Energy.

6. Excess Protein May Contribute to ADHD in Children.

If stomach acid secretion is insufficient, digestive enzymes cannot be activated, resulting in undigested food advancing straight into the intestines.

The quality of food and water determines the health of the entire body. Shinya, Hiromi (2011-10-26).

Cancer is a lifestyle-related disease. Thus, the appearance of cancer somewhere means that most likely there are cancerous cells that have not yet grown into a tumor in other parts of the body... In other words, cancer is not a localized disease that invades only one area of the body. It is a full body disease that affects the body as a whole.

Knowing how to limit the unnecessary depletion of your precious source enzymes is the secret to curing illnesses and living a long and healthy life.

Eat Foods that Contain Plenty of Enzymes. There Is No Fat Worse For Your Body Than Margarine.

Cow's Milk Is Primarily for Calves. That is how nature works. Only humans deliberately take another species' milk, oxidize it and drink it. It goes against natural law.

The Majority of Diseases Are Caused by Habit, Rather than Heredity. Children inherit the good or bad habits of their parents.

Adults who were told by their parents from a young age that they should drink milk every day since it is good for the body are probably still drinking milk—with their parents' words ingrained in their minds. Only by reflecting carefully on our own habits, testing them against the best current nutritional information and taking responsibility can we pass down better health to the next generation.

Shinya, Hiromi (2011-10-26). The Enzyme Factor (Kindle Locations 202- 203). Millichap Books. Kindle Edition.

Learn how you can get a free 30-day supply of Kangen Alkaline water – recommended by Dr. Hiromi Shinya. Watch: http://imanimaat.kangendemo.com

## Appendix K: Mentors Evaluation Form

Your feedback will be used to make revisions to improve the usefulness of this book. Please take a moment to fill this out and return it to us at the address provided below.

### Location:

City _____

State _____

Date of Workshop

_____

—

## Races & Ethnicities Present:

White___

African American/Black____

Hispanic ___

Native American____

Asian____

Pacific Islander___

Other___

## Ages of Youth:

< 9 ___

9-12 ___

13-16 ___

17-20 ___

20 ___

Dr. Imani Ma'at

Number of Youth that participated:

_____


How easy was it to use on a scale of 1-5 with
1 = difficult to 5= very easy _____


In what setting did you use the workbook?
(i.e., school, church, community group)


How did the youth respond to the
workshop?


What did they like the most?

What did they like the least?

Are there particular subjects that you recommend including in next the edition?

If so what subjects?

Other comments?

Dr. Imani Ma'at

Please return to:

Focused Health, LLC
2107 N. Decatur Road, #175,
Decatur, GA 30033

# Healthy Haiku

Dr. Imani Ma'at

## COMMON POETRY TERMS

Alliteration: The repetition of same or similar sounds at the beginning of words. A famous example of alliteration: *Peter Piper picked a peck of pickled peppers!*

Haiku: A Japanese poem composed of three unrhymed lines of five, seven and five syllables. Haiku often reflect on some aspect of nature. Verse: A single metrical line of poetry, or poetry in general (as opposed to prose).

Hyperbole: A figure of speech in which deliberate exaggeration is used for emphasis. Some everyday expressions of hyperbole: *tons of money, waiting for ages, a flood of tears.* Hyperbole is the opposite of Litote.

Litote: A figure of speech in which a positive is stated by negating its opposite. Some examples of litotes: no small victory, not a bad idea, not unhappy. Litotes, which are forms of understatement, is the opposite of hyperbole.

Metaphor: A figure of speech in which two things are compared, usually by saying one thing is another, or by substituting a more descriptive word for the more common or usual word that would be expected. Some examples of metaphors: *the world's a stage, he was a lion in battle, drowning in debt, and a sea of troubles.*

Meter: The arrangement of a line of poetry by the number of syllables and the rhythm of accented (or stressed) syllables.

Onomatopoeia: A figure of speech in which word are used to imitate sound. Examples of onomatopoeia words are buss, hiss, clippety-clop, and tick-tock.

Rhyme: The occurrence of the same or similar sounds at the end of two or more words. When the rhyme occurs in a final stressed syllable, it is said to be masculine: cat/hat, behave/shave, observe/deserve. When the rhyme ends with one of more unstressed syllables , it is said to be feminine: vacation/sensation, reliable/viable. The pattern of rhyme in a stanza or poem is shown usually by using a different for each final sound. In a poem with an *aabba* rhyme scheme, the first, second and fifth lines end in one sound, and the third and fourth lines end in another.

Senryu: A short Japanese poem that is similar to haiku in structure but treats human beings rather than nature, often in a humorous and satiric way.

Simile: A figure of speech in which two things are compared using the word "like" or "as." An example of simile using Langston Hughes poem *Harlem: What happens to a dream deferred?/Does it dry up like a raisin in the sun?*

Stanza: Two or more lines of poetry that together form one of the divisions of a poem. The stanzas of a poem are usually of the same length and follow the same pattern of meter and rhyme.

Source: Glossary of Poetry Terms. Available at:

http://www.infoplease.com/ipa/A0903237.html

Reprinted from Imani Ma'at. (2010)
Healthy Haiku Poetry.
Atlanta: Y.E.S. 4 Health, Inc.

Dr. Imani Ma'at

## ABOUT THE AUTHOR

Dr. Imani Ma'at is a Harvard Educated Acclaimed Author, Award- Winning Health Educator, Researcher, Radio Talk Show Host and Poet with 22 years of experience at the Centers for Disease Control and Prevention (CDC) as Health Scientist & Program Director. She served as the Director of a National Program to Eliminate Health Disparities (REACH 2010) supporting the efforts of community coalitions around the U.S. in the development of new and innovative approaches to chronic diseases and health issues such as diabetes, cancer, HIV/AIDS, heart disease, and breast and cervical cancer.

Dr. Ma'at launched Stepping Into My Power Productions, a subsidiary of Focused Health, LLC. She has created Healthy Haiku Workshops based on her scientifically evaluated and award-winning curriculum that infuses the arts in health education. Her workshops also grew out of her Teen Theater Group (YES 4 Health, Inc.) and through working with mentors, youth and women's organizations over the last 11 years. During workshops, participants learn about health issues and most importantly how to create a powerful lives and environments.

Her mission: To help others to Step Into Their Power in Health and Wellness through Synchronicity at the Individual, Group and Society Levels.

She offers several Exciting Empowerment Programs: (1) Health & Wellness Speaking Engagements and Keynote Presentations; (2) Healthy Haiku Workshops for Youth; (3) Health Coaching for Youth; and (4) Blog Talk Radio Interviews. Clients include schools, universities, corporations, health departments, individuals, women's and youth organizations. She has earned degrees from Mount Holyoke College, M.I.T, Harvard University and Teacher's College of Columbia University.

Dr. Ma'at is available to schedule workshops for children and teens; training for mentors and teachers; Health consulting and motivational speaking engagements for all ages.

To learn more about the Healthy Haiku Method and to purchase other books in the series, visit:

http://www.HealthyHaiku.com

Facebook:

http://facebook.com/healthyhaiku

Twitter: @healthyhaiku

Email: DrImani@DrImaniMaat.com

LinkedIn:

https://www.linkedin.com/in/imanimaat

http://www.DrImaniMaat.com

www.ingramcontent.com/pod-product-compliance
Lightning Source LLC
Chambersburg PA
CBHW062214270326
41930CB00009B/1736